Lasers in Gastroenterology

Lasers in Gastroenterology

International Experiences and Trends

Edited by J. F. Riemann and C. Ell

Foreword by A. G. Hofstetter
Introduction by L. Demling

With Contributions by

S. Bonvoisin
S. G. Bown
A. Chavaillon
M. Classen
F. C. A. Den Hartog Jager
F. Descos
C. Ell
D. Fleischer
F. Frank
H. Fujimura
Y. Fukumoto
J. Giedl
C. Ginsbach
F. Hagenmüller
D. Hashimoto
J. Hochberger
B. Kohler
R. Lambert
G. Lux
N. E. Marcon

E. M. H. Mathus-Vliegen
D. Müller
Y. Okazaki
T. Otani
J. F. Riemann
G. Ries
P. Rutgeerts
G. Sabben
C. Sander
R. Sander
E. Schröder
J. C. Souquet
P. Spinelli
T. Takemoto
I. Tanabe
G. N. J. Tytgat
E. Unsöld
P. J. Valette
G. Vantrappen

92 Figures, 34 Tables

1989
Georg Thieme Verlag   Thieme Medical Publishers, Inc.
Stuttgart · New York   New York

Library of Congress Cataloging in Publication Data

Lasers in gastroenterology / edited by J. F.
Riemann and C. Ell ; foreword by A. G. Hofstetter ;
introduction by L. Demling ; with contributions by
S. Bonvoisin . . . [et al.].
   p. cm.
  Includes bibliographies and index.
  ISBN 0-86577-292-4 (Thieme Medical Publishers)
  1. Gastrointestinal system – Surgery. 2. Lasers
in surgery.
  I. Riemann, Jürgen F. II. Ell, Christian.
III. Bonvoisin, S.
  [DNLM: 1. Gastrointestinal Diseases – radiotherapy.
  2. Laserstherapeutic use. WI 100 C9763]
RD540.C87 1989
617'.43059–dc 19
DNLM/DLC
                               88-36948

Important Note: Medicine is an ever-changing science. Research and clinical experience are continually broadening our knowledge, in particular our knowledge of proper treatment and drug therapy. Insofar as this book mentions any dosage or application, readers may rest assured that the authors, editors and publishers have made every effort to ensure that such references are strictly in accordance with the state of knowledge at the time of production of the book. Nevertheless, every user is requested to carefully examine the manufacturers' leaflets accompanying each drug to check on his own responsibility whether the dosage schedules recommended therein or the contraindications stated by the manufacturers differ from the statements made in the present book. Such examination is particularly important with drugs which are either rarely used or have been newly released on the market.

© 1989 Georg Thieme Verlag, Rüdigerstrasse 14,
D-7000 Stuttgart 30, Germany

Thieme Medical Publishers, Inc., 381 Park Avenue
South, New York, N.Y. 10016

Typesetting by Druckhaus Dörr, Inhaber Adam Götz,
Ludwigsburg (System: Linotype 5/202)
Printed in Germany by Grammlich, Pliezhausen

ISBN 3-13-720501-8 (Georg Thieme Verlag, Stuttgart)
ISBN 0-86577-292-4 (Thieme Medical Publishers, Inc.
New York)   2 3 4 5 6

Foreword

The multiplicity of the laser opens new and unexpected possibilities in diagnostics and therapy in the different fields of medicine. With this optimistic declaration, we have to consider that we are still at the beginning of this new technology, which means that we have to expect not only success but also failure. Important things are already being done by the laser in the field of tumor destruction. New possibilities are shown by the results in endoscopic stone destruction executed in the recent past. Clinical advantages in the treatment of endoscopic bleeding aided by the neodymium : YAG laser were again and again described in gastroenterology. Before us lies the wide field of angioplasty, for which we have still to prove the superiority of the laser.

Gastroenterology, like neurosurgery and urology, is one of the fields that is well suited to the laser. Therefore, it seems appropriate that experienced persons using the laser in gastroenterology take the trouble to write a book about their experiences.

As present President of the German Society for Laser Medicine and as President of the International Society for Laser Surgery and Medicine, I welcome this activity and I wish complete success for the work.

Lübeck, Fall 1988

Prof. Dr. A. G. Hofstetter

Preface

Photocoagulation by laser beam has become established as one of the important methods among gastroenterologic techniques in recent years. Whereas treating gastrointestinal bleeding used to be its most common indication, laser therapy is now mostly used in the treatment of cancers. National and international experiences have shown promising results and have been reported at many congresses, the last of which was the World Congress of Gastroenterology in Sao Paulo, Brasil, in 1986. We have tried to collect all different worldwide activities and experiences and to publish them in a single volume. This book not only deals with the progress made so far, it also points out aspects, that have yet to be realized or that are already being realized in many institutions, for example, photodynamic techniques.

We have been successful in engaging many well-known international experts to participate in this book, which was intended to focus on important aspects in laser therapy and to acquaint a large number of persons with them.

With such a new technique, it is inevitable that different investigators gain different experiences and opinions about the technique. We deliberately want to present a broad range of, in part, controversial opinions in this book. We are thankful to all participants for their discipline in writing their manuscripts.

We hope that this book shall quickly find many readers; the level and the extent of knowledge in this field have expanded tremendously in the last 2 years, so that we expect a second edition to become necessary soon, in which we hope to show that in certain controversial aspects a broader consensus has been reached.

Ludwigshafen and Erlangen,
Fall 1988

J. F. Riemann
C. Ell

Addresses

Bown, S. G., Dr.
National Medical Laser Centre
Faculty of Clinical Sciences
University College London
5 University Street
London WC1E 6JJ

Ell, C., Priv.-Doz. Dr. med.
Med. Klinik I mit Poliklinik
der Universität Erlangen-Nürnberg
Krankenhausstraße 12
D-8520 Erlangen

Fleischer, D., M. D.
Division of Gastroenterology
Georgetown University Hospital
3800 Reservoir Road
Washington, D. C. 20007 U. S. A.

Frank, F., Dr.
MBB-Medizintechnik GmbH
Applikationsforschung
PO Box 80 11 68
D-8000 München 80

Giedl, J., Priv.-Doz. Dr. med.
Abteilung für Klinische Pathologie
Chirurgische Universitätsklinik
Maximiliansplatz
D-8520 Erlangen

Hagenmüller, F., Priv.-Doz. Dr. med.
II. Medizinische Klinik und Poliklinik
der Technischen Universität München
Ismaninger Straße 22
D-8000 München 80

Hashimoto, D., M. D.
Second Department of Surgery
School of Medicine
Tokyo University
7-3-1, Hongo, Bunkyo-Ku
Tokyo, Japan

Hochberger, J., Dr.
Med. Klinik I mit Poliklinik
der Universität Erlangen-Nürnberg
Krankenhausstraße 12
D-8520 Erlangen

Kohler, B., Dr.
Medizinische Klinik C
Klinikum der Stadt Ludwigshafen
Bremserstraße 79
D-6700 Ludwigshafen

Lambert, R., Prof. Dr.
Hôpital Edouard-Herriot
Service d'hepato-gastroenterologie
Place d'Arsonval
F-69374 Lyon

Marcon, N. E., Dr.
Division of Gastroenterology
The Wellesley Hospital
160 Wellesley Street East
Toronto, Ontario M4Y 1J3
Canada

Mathus-Vliegen, E. M. H., Dr.
Department of Gastroenterology-Hepatology
Academic Medical Center
Meibergdreef 9
NL-1105 AZ Amsterdam

Riemann, J. F., Prof. Dr.
Direktor der Medizinischen Klinik C
Klinikum der Stadt Ludwigshafen
Bremserstraße 79
D-6700 Ludwigshafen

Rutgeerts, P., M. D. Ass. Prof.
Department of Medicine
Division of Gastroenterology
University Hospital Gasthuisberg
B-3000 Leuven

Sander, R., Dr.
Städtisches Krankenhaus
München-Harlaching
I. Medizinische Abteilung
Sanatoriumsplatz 2
D-8000 München 90

Schröder, E.,
Meditec – Aesculap
Obere Bergstraße 3
D-8501 Heroldsberg

Spinelli, P., Prof. Dr.
Divisione Endoscopia
Instituto Nazionale Tumori
V. Venezian 1
I-20133 Milano

Takemoto, T., Dr.
The First Department of Internal Medicine
Yamaguchi University
School of Medicine
Ube City, Yamaguchi Pref., 755
Japan

Tytgat, G. N. J., Prof. Dr.
Department of Gastroenterology-Hepatology
Academic Medical Center
Meibergdreef 9
NL-1105 AZ Amsterdam

Unsöld, E., Dr.
Zentrales Laserlabor der Gesellschaft für
Strahlen- und Umweltforschung (GSF)
Ingolstädter Landstraße 1
D-8042 Neuherberg

Contents

Future Trends

General Considerations

Introduction

L. Demling

Laser light is a highly efficient form of energy which was discovered in 1960 by Theodore Maiman. It can be beamed on target in any desired wavelength and depth of penetration, and in exactly defined doses. As for every other energy, laser energy can be converted into other energy forms. In gastroenterology, in particular, the laser beam also exercises a thermal action, producing coagulation, carbonization, and vaporization. Thus, laser therapy can achieve hemostasis and prevent hemorrhage besides destroying stenosing or nonstenosing tumors. Laser-supported photodynamic therapy using hematoporphyrin derivates is a valuable aid in fighting cancer. These derivatives are stored selectively in tumors and stimulated by fluorescence, producing cytotoxic oxygen and hydroxyl radicals in the tumor. Undesirable tissue structures can also be destroyed by laser-induced photoablation. This uses high electromagnetic field strengths to disrupt molecular structures without an intermediate thermal stage. In photoacoustic interaction, which uses a similar energy range, laser light produces thermal, usually periodic, shock waves, destroying material of poor elasticity, such as concrements. In this manner gallstones can be broken down when brought into contact with laser light conductors.

We speak of photodisruption or optical breakdown if the conversion of light into high temperatures yields ionized plasma, which on being heated again produces a miniexplosion. To achieve this photomechanical effect, laser light must be broken down into high energy and hence extremely short impulses. Photodisruption can also be used to destroy stones.

Laser light was an immediate success in gastroenterology because highly sophisticated endoscopes were already available as guides for directing the laser beam on-target via flexible thin light conductors requiring only slight resetting and conversion.

Laser in gastroenterology signifies not only hemostasis, tumor treatment, removal of stenoses, and breaking down of concrements, but also – an important aspect indeed – sparing of organ structures not directly involved in disease. Laser light, if properly adapted both qualitatively and quantitatively to the therapeutic goal, can replace surgery in a number of fields. It is, in fact, in line with an old medical axiom: faster, safer, easier (on the patient): *cito, tuto, jucunde.*

Fundamental Principles

Basic Physics and Biophysics

F. Frank

Physical Principles

The term "laser" is an acronym for light amplification by stimulated emission of radiation. The possibility of laser action was first suggested by Albert Einstein (6) in 1917. In 1954, Charles H. Townes (12) built the forerunner of the laser, a microwave amplifier, to which he gave the name "maser", an acronym for microwave amplification by stimulated emission of radiation. At about the same time, Basov and Prokhorov (1) independently produced a maser of their own. In 1958, Townes collaborated with Schawlow (23) on a historic paper that laid the theoretical foundation for the laser, then referred to as an optical maser. All of this preliminary work culminated in 1960 when Theodore H. Maiman (18) constructed the first working laser using a rod of crystalline ruby excited by a coaxial helical flash lamp. In rather rapid succession, other lasers were built, notably, the helium-neon (He-Ne) by Javan, et al. (15) in 1961; the argon ion by Bridges (3) in 1964; the carbon dioxide (CO_2) by Patel (21) in 1964; and the neodymium:yttrium-aluminum-garnet (Nd:YAG) by Geusic, et al. (11) in 1964.

The expression "light amplification by stimulated emission of radiation" states the goal of light amplification; stimulated emission of radiation is the means of achieving it. The terms "light", "amplification", and "radiation" are well known. To explain "stimulated emission", it is necessary to know something about absorption and emission.

Absorption

According to the atomic model by Bohr, the electrons in an atomic system revolve in separate levels around the nucleus, which is composed of protons and neutrons. Each of these levels corresponds to a certain energy. If there is an interaction between light photons with the orbital electrons, the light energy is absorbed and an electron is able to change from one level to the next. This process is called absorption (Fig. 1).

Spontaneous Emission

Having absorbed energy in this way, the atom will spontaneously return to a lower energy state after a while. Normally, an electron can stay in an upper level only if the lower level is completely occupied. When the electrons return to the lower energy trajectory, if this decay is radiative, a photon with a wavelength that is proportional to the difference in energy levels is emitted. This process is called spontaneous emission (Fig. 1).

Stimulated Emission

In the process of stimulated emission, a photon of a specific wavelength hits an atom in the excited state and causes the electrons to decay to a lower energy state faster than would occur spontaneously. In this case, the incident radiation and the emitted photon travel in the same direction, are in phase, and are of exactly the same wavelength. One photon leads to the emission of a second similar one (Fig. 1).

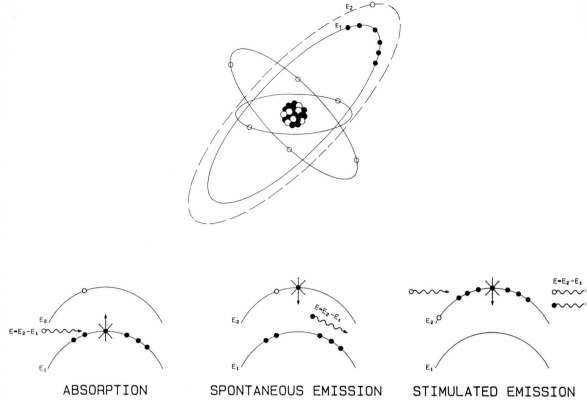

ABSORPTION   SPONTANEOUS EMISSION   STIMULATED EMISSION

Fig. **1** Diagram of an atom and the characteristics of absorption, spontaneous emission, and stimulated emission of a photon.

Light Amplification

A light amplifier is a lasing medium, that is, a material capable of stimulated emission, enclosed between two parallel mirrors, the so-called optical resonator. The lasing medium, which may be ions, atoms, or molecules in a solid, liquid, or gas phase, is excited by a pump source that uses light, electrical, or chemical energy. In the excited active laser medium photons are emitted spontaneously in all directions. A good laser medium remains in the excited state for a relatively long period of time. The small population of photons emitted along the axis of the laser resonator will create a cascade of photons. Reflection of photons by the mirrors amplifies the number of photons generated by stimulated emission. One of the mirrors is partially transmitting, which permits some of the photons to be emitted from the laser resonator, creating a beam of laser light (Fig. **2**).

Properties of Laser Light

Laser light has certain characteristics that distinguish it from ordinary light:

– All emitted photons are of the same wavelengths; therefore, the beam is *monochromatic*.
– All the waves, i.e., the photons, are in phase, so the beam will be *temporally coherent*.
– All the photons travel in the same direction, so the beam will be spatially coherent or collimated with very *low divergence*.

Because of these properties, the beam can be focused to achieve high energy densities,

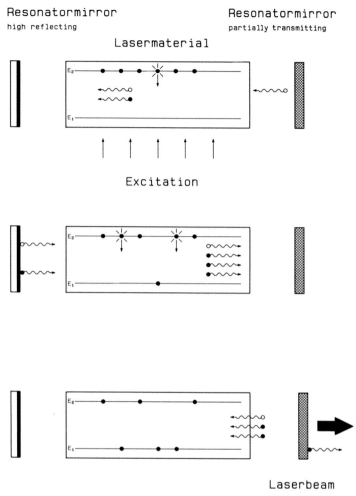

Fig. **2**   Principle of laser with the optical resonator, excitation of the
laser medium, and light amplification.

making precise working with the laser beam possible.

Laser light can be focused to form very small diameter beams. Focusing the laser beam can increase its intensity by many orders of magnitude. For example, the average power density of sunlight is 0.1 W/cm², whereas power densities of 100,000 W/cm² are easily obtained with surgical laser systems. Striking a match produces an energy of 200 J (W) of incoherent light. With only 1 J of coherent light from a ruby laser it is possible, by focusing with a simple lens, to drill a hole through metal.

By using different lasing media, laser systems with different emitted wavelengths can be constructed beginning in the ultraviolet region at about 200 nm and reaching into the infrared up to a wavelength of 10 μm (Fig. **3**).

In the region of wavelengths between 300 nm and 2.2 μm it is possible to transmit laser light in very thin but still mechanically robust quartz glass fibers (0.2 to 0.6 mm in diameter) on the basis of successive total internal reflection. This is one reason why the Nd:YAG laser is currently used in gastroenterologic endoscopy.

Laser systems differ also with regard to

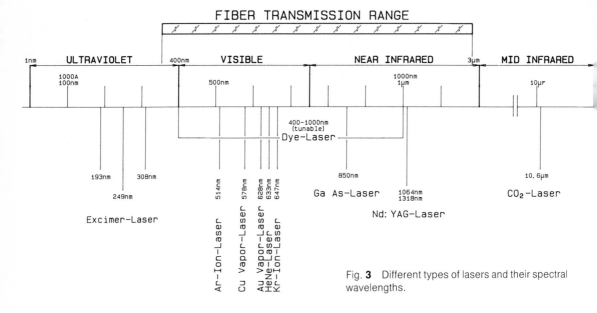

Fig. **3**   Different types of lasers and their spectral wavelengths.

duration and power of the emitted laser radiation. In *continuous wave lasers* (cw mode) with power outputs of up to 10^3 W, the lasing medium is excited continuously. With *pulsed lasers,* excitation is effected in a single pulse or in on-line pulses *(free-running-mode)*. Peak powers of 10^5 W can be developed for a duration of 10 ms to 100 μs. Storing the excitation energy and releasing it suddenly *(q-switch mode* or *mode locking)* leads to a peak power increase of up to 10^{10} to 10^{12} W and a pulse duration of 100 ns to 10 ps (Fig. **4**).

Biophysical Considerations

When considering the interaction between laser light and biologic tissues, the physical parameters of the biologic object must be re-

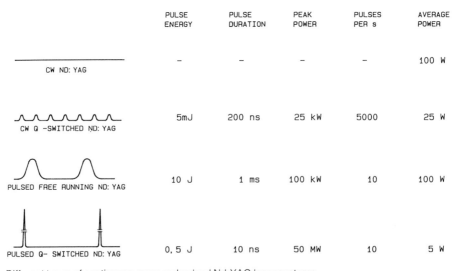

	PULSE ENERGY	PULSE DURATION	PEAK POWER	PULSES PER s	AVERAGE POWER
CW ND: YAG	–	–	–	–	100 W
CW Q –SWITCHED ND: YAG	5mJ	200 ns	25 kW	5000	25 W
PULSED FREE RUNNING ND: YAG	10 J	1 ms	100 kW	10	100 W
PULSED Q– SWITCHED ND: YAG	0,5 J	10 ns	50 MW	10	5 W

Fig. **4**   Different types of continuous wave and pulsed Nd:YAG laser systems.

lated to the parameters of the laser light. The degree and extent of the effect depend on the properties of the tissue, which are determined by the structure, water content, and blood circulation, i. e., absorption, scattering, reflection, thermal conductivity, heat capacity, and density, as well as on the geometry of the laser beam, i. e., its power density, energy content, and wavelength (Fig. 5).

Depending on the duration of the laser irradiation on the tissue *(interaction time)*, on the one hand, and on the laser irradiance in surface or volume interaction with tissue *(effective power density)*, on the other hand, three types of tissue interaction can be distinguished.

– Photochemical effects (10 s to 1000 s; 10^{-3} to 1 W/cm^2)
– Photothermal effects (1 ms to 100 s; 1 to 10^6 W/cm^2)
– Photoionizing effects (10 ps to 100 ns; 10^8 to 10^{12} W/cm^2)

Photochemical Effects

In extremely long interaction times and low-power densities, photochemical transformation occurs by absorption of light with no primary heating of the tissue.

The most important example is *photosensitized oxidation*. The combined use of laser light and an injected photosensitizer, today mainly hematoporphyrin derivates (HPD), ini-

tiate a cytotoxic process. Most of the tissue is destroyed after excitation of the photosensitizer by laser light. The stimulated sensitizer undergoes a series of intramolecular chemical reactions that lead to the oxidation of various cellular components (5). The fact that the residence time of HPD in pathologic tissue is longer than in healthy tissue permits selective tumor eradication. In photodynamic therapy, use is made of argon pumped *dye lasers* (1 W at 630 nm, cw), and *gold vapor lasers* (10 W at 628 nm, pulsed). HPD has significant side effects. Other photosensitizers for different types of tissue have to be developed.

Biostimulation mainly for wound healing or pain relief belongs to this field, too. Systematic studies have not yet given reasonable explanations for the clinically observed improvements (19). Use is made of the *He-Ne laser* (1 to 5 mW at 633 nm) and *gallium arsenide laser diodes* (5 mW at 850 nm).

Photothermal Effects

With decreasing interaction time and higher power density, the transition to photothermally induced effects begins. The main surgical applications for lasers are based on the conversion of laser light into heat. This thermal effect is broadly applied in surgery for tissue removal and tissue coagulation with sealing of vessels and lymphatics and for tissue welding.

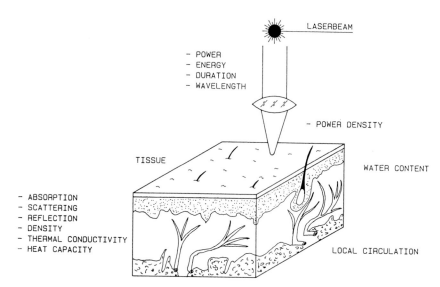

Fig. **5** Diagram of the parameters that determine the effects of laser light in tissue.

The *thermal denaturation* of tissue takes place approximately as follows. To a large extent both the structure and the function of living cells are determined by a wide variety of proteins. These macromolecules have a highly ordered structure, whose energy is stable at body temperature. If the temperature is increased locally to about 50°C or more, a certain percentage of the molecules pass into an energy activated state from which an irreversible transition into the denaturated state takes place. When this happens, the protein molecule loses its spatial arrangement to some extent, and with it, its power to function in the cell. Depending on the nature of the irradiated tissue, individual thermolabile enzymes may play the leading role in the tissue reaction. There then follows a delayed tissue necrosis, although little or no structural damage to the tissue can be seen immediately after the irradiation.

The degree and the extent of the thermal action depend, on the one hand, on the optical and thermal properties of the tissue and, on the other hand, on the laser beam geometry and energy of the incident light.

The most important optical parameter is the wavelength-dependent *absorption* of biologic molecules. Since the building blocks of living systems, amino acids, proteins, and nucleic acids, despite their great variety, are made up of only a few basic elements, some few fundamental rules can be formulated for the absorption of optical radiation. The main absorption of biologic molecules occurs within the range of wavelengths shorter than approximately 280 nm. The far more molecule-specific vibrational and rotational absorption bands are all in the range of wavelengths longer than 1 μm. Visible laser radiation is hardly absorbed by biologic material. One of the most important exceptions to this rule is the hemoglobin in the red blood corpuscles, and melanin, which is stored as a pigment in the skin and also in large quantities in the pigment epithelium of the retina. A strong absorption in the green spectrum occurs in both substances. The high water content (60%) of most tissue leads to an extensive absorption of infrared radiation. This leads to very efficient energy transfer and heating of the tissue when irradiating with lasers of these wavelengths.

In addition to absorption, *scattering* must be considered as a further optical tissue para-

meter. Tissue is a highly structured medium, so that directed optical radiation is completely altered in its spatial distribution due to reflection, refraction, and diffraction. This scattering effect mainly comes into play when absorption is weak.

The thermal properties of tissue, the *heat capacity* and conductivity, can be taken in the first approximation to be the same as those of water. However, estimation of the spread of the energy by *thermal conductivity* is often very difficult when tissue layers of strongly differing structure and complicated geometry are involved, such as the stomach wall, the retina, and the bladder wall, or when blood vessels give rise to a very non homogeneous removal of energy due to the usually irregular blood flow.

The temperature increase and temperature distribution in tissue exposed to laser radiation depend on the energy absorbed by the volume of tissue and on the thermal properties of the tissue. The thermal properties determine the temperature increase and the consequent change in temperature distribution after the exposure. According to the temperature in the tissue, changes such as discoloration, *coagulation*, shrinkage, *carbonization*, and *vaporization* occur. In this process it should be noted that coagulation, unlike vaporization, consumes no additional heat. Vaporization is associated with heat consumption, but despite continued exposure, the tissue temperature does not increase during the phase transition (Fig. 6).

The choice of wavelength determines the depth of penetration according to the kind of tissue and thus influences the interplay between the different tissue reactions. With the CO_2 *laser* (up to 100 W at 10.6 μm), absorption by tissue is the strongest and scattering is negligible. The light energy is, therefore, completely converted into heat at the tissue surface. For this reason, the CO_2 laser as a cutting tool with a small depth of penetration is well suited for removing tissue.

The absorption of *argon laser* radiation (up to 10 W, 488 nm, 514 nm) is weaker than that of the CO_2 laser radiation. The scattering of the argon laser emission is not pronounced. The penetration is limited due to the selective absorption in hemoglobin and melanin. Its application is thus restricted to indications in which removal of the tissue with simultaneous limited coagulation is desired.

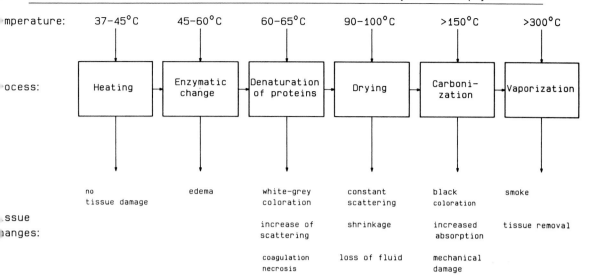

Temperature:	37–45°C	45–60°C	60–65°C	90–100°C	>150°C	>300°C

Process:

Heating	Enzymatic change	Denaturation of proteins	Drying	Carboni-zation	Vaporization

Tissue changes:

no tissue damage	edema	white–grey coloration	constant scattering	black coloration	smoke
		increase of scattering	shrinkage	increased absorption	tissue removal
		coagulation necrosis	loss of fluid	mechanical damage	

Fig. **6**   Thermal tissue alterations after laser irradiation.

The *Nd:YAG laser* emits light in the near infrared range (up to 100 W at 1064 nm and up to 30 W at 1318 nm). At the wavelength of 1064 nm, absorption in tissue is very low. Scattering is therefore very pronounced, resulting in uniform distribution of the radiation in the tissue.

Slow heating of a large tissue volume around the point of impingement of the radiation occurs, followed by deep coagulation that progresses slowly. Finally, protoplasm vaporizes at the tissue surface, leading to marked shrinking, although the tissue surface itself is hardly damaged. The shrinking of the tissue combined with uniform coagulation results in a sealing of blood and lymph vessels. Arteries of up to 2 mm and veins of up to 3 mm in diameter are closed rapidly and reliably.

Owing to the shrinkage effect, the coagulation layer causes mechanical compression of the vessels, which results in hemostasis. The sealing off of the bleeding source is assisted by the gluelike consistency of the denatured tissue.

With Nd:YAG laser irradiation at 1064 nm, the coagulation volume or damage zone increases according to intensity, then carbonization occurs at the surface, and the tissue is vaporized and removed (10). These are further reasons that have led to the application of the Nd:YAG laser in gastroenterology for the endoscopic treatment of tumors, stenoses, and control of hemorrhage (16, 17).

The absorption coefficient of water and saline is approximately ten times higher using the Nd:YAG laser at a wavelength of 1318 nm than at 1064 nm. A more efficient conversion of energy into heat occurs in tissue at 1318 nm. The extinction coefficient (which depends on scattering and absorption) in blood at 1318 nm is only one-third that at 1064 nm (26). This results in less heat dissipation by blood and deeper penetration in tissue at 1318 nm.

Particularly in tissue with a high water content, a marked loosening of the necrotic tissue is obtained with laser light of the 1318 nm wavelength, resulting in a certain ablative effect with effective power densities of up to 30 kW/cm². However, it is by no means to be compared with the well-known precise incision obtained with a 10.6 μm CO_2 laser. Unlike the CO_2 laser incision, tissue ablation with the Nd:YAG laser at 1318 nm is distinguished by a clear and effective coagulation zone along the borders of the incision. With a significantly lower effective power density and an interaction time of 0.1 s, the resulting sharply defined coagulation can be used for tissue welding (9, 22, 24).

An additional thermal effect is produced by using flash lamp pumped free-running mode Nd:YAG lasers (2 J with 10 ms at

1064 nm) or pulsed dye lasers (100 mJ with 200 µs between 450 and 600 nm) for stone destruction. This thermal lithotriptic effect is explained by heat conduction to the water in the microcavities of the stone. The high vaporization pressure leads to the fragmentation of the stone (4, 7). This procedure is of limited clinical significance, since the high temperatures produced can damage neighboring organs.

Photoionizing Effects

When a power density of 10^7 W/cm^2 is exceeded, *nonlinear effects* result. The high irradiance generates strong electric fields, which lead to a *dissociation* or *ionization* of the material involved. Thus, laser light is converted into kinetic energy.

The high photon density causes an increased absorption and a direct nonthermal breakdown of the intramolecular bonds. This feature is known as photoablation and has been exploited to produce precise ($> 50 \, \mu m$) non-necrotic cuts by using argon fluoride, krypton fluoride, xenon chloride excimer lasers (10^8 W/cm^2 with 10 ns at 193, 249, and 308 nm).

The focusing of even shorter high-peak power laser pulses creates power densities (10^{10} W/cm^2 for nanosecond pulses and 10^{12} W/cm^2 for picosecond pulses), which generate such powerful electric fields (10^6 to 10^7 V/cm) that spontaneous ionization of free electrons and ionized atoms *(plasma)* is induced. When a certain degree of ionization has been reached, an increase in temperature of the plasma follows. Thereupon, the plasma undergoes a sudden expansion accompanied by a mechanical-acoustic shock wave. The shock wave ruptures the tissue structure *(photodisruption)* or disintegrates the targeted material *(photofragmentation)*.

Use is made of those ionizing effects in ophthalmology in microsurgical interventions within the eye without any damage to the healthy anatomic structures. Using pulsed q-switched Nd:YAG lasers or pulsed dye lasers and coupling high-pulse energies (80 mJ with 10 ns at 1064 nm or 60 mJ with 1.5 µs at 590 nm, respectively) into flexible glass fibers, it is possible to smash gallstones in vitro (8, 25), and to fragment kidney and ureter stones in patients (13, 14).

Laser Application in Gastroenterology

Due to the biophysical interactions outlined, the application of the laser in gastroenterology at present can be summarized as follows:

– Destruction of tumors, ablation of stenosing tissue, and treatment of hemorrhages with the cw Nd:YAG laser
– Management of tumors with dye lasers in combination with HPD
– Fragmentation of gallstones with the aid of free-running Nd:YAG lasers, pulsed dye lasers, or q-switched Nd:YAG lasers.

References

1 Basov, N G, Prokhorov, A M: J. Exp. Theoret. Phys. (USSR), 27. 431, 1954
2 Boulnois, J-L: Photophysical processes in recent medical laser developments: A review. Laser Med. Sci. 1: 47, 1986
3 Bridges W B: Laser oscillation in singly ionized argon in the visible spectrum. Appl. Phys. Lett. 4: 128, 1964
4 Deutsch TF, Oseroff AR: New medical uses of lasers: A survey. Baltimore: Proc CLEO 1985: paper WF 3
5 Dougherty TJ: Photoradiation Therapy – Clinical and Drug Advances, Porphyrin Photosensitisation. Plenum Press, New York 1983
6 Einstein A: On the quantum theory of radiation. Physikalische Z, 18: 121, 1917
7 Ell C, Hochberger J, Müller D, Zirngibl H, Giedl J, Lux G, Demling L: Laser lithotripsy of gallstone by means of a pulsed neodymium-YAG laser – in vitro and animal experiments. Endoscopy 18: 92, 1986
8 Ell C, Wondrazek F, Frank F, Hochberger J, Lux G, Demling L: Laser-induced shockwave lithotripsy of gallstones. Endoscopy 18: 95, 1986
9 Frank F, Beck OJ, Hessel S, Keiditsch E: Comparative investigations of the effects of the Nd:YAG laser at 1.06 µm and 1.32 µm on tissue. Lasers Surg Med 6: 546, 1986
10 Frank F, Hofstetter AG, Keiditsch E: Experimental investigation and new instrumentation for Nd:YAG laser treatment in urology. In: Bellina JH (ed): Gynecologic Laser Surgery. Plenum Press, New York 1981 (p. 345)
11 Geusic, JE, Marcos HW, Van Uitert LG: Laser oscillations in Nd:doped yttrium aluminum, yttrium gallium, and gadolinium garnets. Appl. Phys. Lett 4: 182, 1964
12 Gordon, JP, Zeiger HJ, Townes CH: Molecular microwave oscillator and new hyperfine structure in the microwave spectrum of NH$_3$. Phys Rev 95: 282, 1954

13 Hofstetter A, Frank F, Keiditsch E, Wondrazek F: Intracorporale, laserinduzierte Stoßwellen-Lithotripsie. Laser Med. Surg 1: 155, 1985

14 Hofstetter A, Schmeller N, Pensel J, Arnholdt H, Frank F, Wondrazek F: Harnstein-Lithotripsie mit laserinduzierten Stoßwellen. Fortschr Med, 35: 32, 1986

15 Javan A, Bennett WR Jr, Herriot DR: Population inversion and continuous optical maser oscillation in a gas discharge containing a helium-neon mixture. Phys. Rev. Lett 6: 106, 1961

16 Kiefhaber P, Kiefhaber K, Huber F, Nath G: Neodymium-YAG laser application for stenosing carcinomas and neoplastic sessile polyps of the gastrointestinal tract. In: Waidelich W (ed): Optoelectronic in der Medizin – Optoelectronic in Medicine 1983. Proceedings of the 6th International Congress Laser 83 Optoelectronic; Springer, Berlin 1984 (p. 75)

17 Kiefhaber P, Nath G, Moritz K: Endoscopical control of massive gastrointestinal hemorrhage by irradiation with a high-power neodymium-YAG laser. Prog Surg 15: 140, 1977

18 Maiman TH: Phys Rev Lett 4: 564, 1960

19 Mester E: Laser application in promoting wound healing. In: Koebner HK (ed): Lasers in Medicine. Wiley, Chichester 1980 (p. 83)

20 Müller GJ, Berlien P, Scholz C: Der Laser in der Medizin. Umschau 1986; 233

21 Patel CKN: Selective excitation through vibrational energy transfer and optical maser action in N_2–CO_2. Phys. Rev Lett 13: 617, 1964

22 Sander R, Pösl H, Strobel M, Unsöld E, Frank F, Spuhler A: Nd:YAG Laser in der Gastroenterologie – Erste Ergebnisse experimenteller und klinischer Studien mit der 1,32 μm Wellenlänge. Laser 2: 167, 1986

23 Schawlow AL, Townes CH: Infrared and optical masers. Phys Rev 112: 1940, 1958

24 Schober R, Ulrich F, Sander T, Dürselen H, Hessel S: Laser-induced alteration of collagen substructure allows microsurgical tissue welding. Science 232: 1421, 1986

25 Simon W, Hering P: Laserinduzierte Stoßwellen-lithotripsie an Nieren- und Gallensteinen (in vitro). Laser Optoelektronik 1: 33, 1987

26 Stokes LF, Auth D, Tanaka J, Gray L, Gulacsik C: Biomedical utility of 1.32 μm Nd:YAG laser radiation. IEEE Trans Biomed Eng 28: 297, 1981

Current Laser Systems

E. Unsöld

The laser is a source of electromagnetic radiation "with unique properties" so far not observed in nature (35). When applying this "completely artificial" radiation to man for medical purposes, a nearly innumerable quantity of factors has to be taken into account. These factors depend on basic physics and medicine as well as on clinical details and demands and on the human nature of the patient and physician. All these factors contribute to what might be called in a broad sense a laser-medical system.

In the following, this term will be restricted to the technical components of the laser-related hardware, which is necessary for an advantageous and safe application of laser and in comparison with conventional methods.

In general, several auxiliary and subsystems are needed to generate laser radiation, guide it to the operation site and finally to the area to be treated, and to control the beam and its quality with respect to power, time behavior, focalization, and safety (11, 37). Thus, the total laser system comprises the following components (Fig. **1**):

– Laser head
– Power supply
– Cooling device
– Light control and shutter system with
– Remote control (optional)
– Radiation transfer system with applicator and beam shaper
– Power meter and dose sensor
– Safety installations and interlock circuits

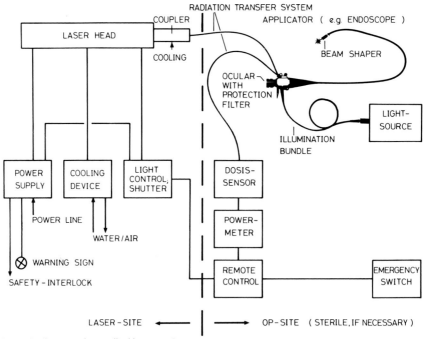

Fig. **1** Schematic diagram of a medical laser system.

Depending on the size and type of laser, some of these components may be integrated into one unit to make transportation easy between different operation sites (23). For other applications, it might be practical to separate these components and even install them in different rooms (21, 22). A central laser unit connected to a distribution system, guiding the radiation to different sites, is also possible (34). Practicability, reliability, and effectiveness, also with respect to costs, should determine the decision.

The *laser head* contains the power laser itself, which delivers radiation according to the

Table **1** Current Laser Systems

Laser Type	Wavelength	Max. Output Power	Electric Power	Cooling	Further Requirements	Remarks
Thermal laser interaction with tissue						
Nd:YAG	1064 nm	150 W	12–20 kW	Air or H_2O 10 l/min	–	Transmission through flexible fibers
Nd:YAG	1318 nm	40 W	12–20 kW	Air or H_2O 10 l/min	–	Transmission through flexible fibers
Argon ion	488; 515 nm	20 W	85 kW	25 l/min H_2O	–	Expensive plasma tube replacement
CO_2	10.6 μm	150 W	3–10 kW	Air or H_2O 5–10 l/min	Gas mixture 0–10 l/h	Transmission through articulated arm
Photochemical laser interaction with photosensitized tissue						
Gold vapor	628 nm	10 W	7 kW	H_2O 4 l/min	Au 0.1 g/h He 1.0 l/h	10 ns pulses at 7–10 kHz repetition frequency
Dye, Ar Laser-pumped	630 nm	4 W	100 kW	H_2O 30 l/min	–	Low efficiency, high prime and running costs
Laser excitation of fluorescence from photosensitized tissue for diagnostic purposes						
Krypton ion	407; 413; 415; 468; 476; 483 nm	0.1–1 W	90 kW	H_2O 28 l/min	–	Computer-controlled switching of wavelength

Laser Type	Wavelenght	Pulse Energy	Pulse Duration	Repetition Frequency	Remarks
Laser-generated shockwaves in concrements					
Dye*	430–750 nm	100 mJ	200 μs	10–100 Hz	Flash lamp-pumped
Dye	590 nm	60 mJ	1.5 μs	10–100 Hz	Flash lamp-pumped
Nd:YAG	1064 nm	2 J	10 ms	10–200 Hz	Flash lamp-pumped
Nd:YAG	1064 nm	80 mJ	10 ns	10–200 Hz	Q-switch
Ablative laser photodecomposition of tissue					
Excimer** ArF	193 nm		20–150 W	quasi continuous-ly 750–1000 Hz	
KrF	248 nm				
XeCl	308 nm				
XeF	351 nm				

See also chapter by Frank and by Ell et al.
* (15, 20), ** (14, 15)

physical and medical demands. This radiation is characterized by the parameters: wavelength (in the ultraviolet (UV), visible, or infrared (IR) wavelength range), power (milliwatt to several hundred watt), time behavior of emission (continuous wave (cw) to picosecond pulses with repetition frequencies up to several kHz), and beam divergence (mrad range, equals approximately 0.06°). It is obvious that this wide range of parameters would demand a broad variety of lasers. However, for practical medical application, especially in gastroenterology, only a few types are in use; several others are promising for the near future.

In Table **1** the current laser types are listed according to their modes of application. These can be classified as follows:

- Thermal laser interaction, the majority of all laser applications (4)
- Photochemical laser interaction with photosensitized tissue, the basis of photodynamic therapy (PDT) (36)
- Fluorescence excitation, a broad field for analytic and diagnostic methods (2, 32)
- Shock wave generation for lithotripsy (15) (see also chapters by Frank and by Ell et al.)
- Ablative photodecomposition (16, 17)

The group "biostimulating effects" has been omitted in Table **1** because of its lack of

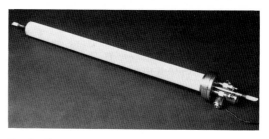

Fig. **2**   Plasma tube of a 20 W argon ion laser (Photo: Spectra Physics, Inc., Mountain View).

relevance to this volume. Several working mechanisms are controversial, but reliable double-blind studies are not known (12).

Table 2 gives some data about lasers, which, due to their physical properties, are promising for future developments, but at present are only in an experimental state.

Gas and metal vapor lasers are directly, electrically pumped via electrodes attached to the laser tube, which contains the laser medium. Figure **2** shows an argon ion laser tube in a metal-ceramic construction. Solid-state and dye lasers are optically pumped via arc or flash lamps or even another gas laser. Thus, the laser head has also to contain these

Table **2**   Future Laser Systems

Laser Type	Wavelength	Output (at present) Power	Energy	Remarks	Reference
Cu vapor	511;578 nm	50 W		Quasi-continuously Dye-pumping, shock waves	18
Ti:Al$_2$O$_3$	680–1100 nm		0.3 J	Tunable	7
Semiconductor	0.7–1.3 μm	2 W (kW-pulse-peak)			10, 14
Alexandrit	720–790 nm	50 W	0.4 J	Quasi-continuously	19
Er:YAG	1.66–1.73 μm 2.73–2.92 μm		1 J	Quasi-continuously	25
Ho	2.1 μm	35 W			24
CO	5–6 μm	20 W			24
CO$_2$	9.24–9.58 μm	50 W		Tunable	28
Free-electron	μ–mm		20 J	500–750 keV electron beam accelerator necessary	1, 5, 27

elements and the corresponding mounts and optical components. The dimensions and weight of laser heads range from hand-held models of carbon dioxide (CO_2) laser with a few watts of output to about $200 \times 35 \times 35 \, cm^3$ ($L \times W \times H$) and 80 kg for a 9 W gold vapor laser.

Pulse shaping Q-switch, wavelength selector (3), or simple shutter elements have to be positioned intracavity into the power laser.

For UV or IR laser another low-power pilot laser, usually a helium-neon laser with red or optionally green emission is provided to emit collinearly to the invisible power beam for its precise adjustment and aiming.

The *power supply* provides the electrical power required either to pump a laser directly by a gas discharge or to operate the optical pumping source (arc lamp, gas laser, or capacitor-driven flash lamp). The output power of a laser can, to a certain amount, be preset or stabilized by an appropriate regulation of the pump power or the electrical input (see light control, etc.). Depending on the output power of the laser and its efficiency, the power consumption of current laser systems ranges between 3 kW for a 60 W CO_2 laser and 100 kW for a 4 W laser-pumped dye laser.

The efficiency, i.e., the coefficient of radiation output to electrical input power, of most lasers is very poor. For the two lasers mentioned before, it amounts to 0.02 and 4×10^{-5}, or 2% and 0.004%, respectively. Only a small amount of the primary energy is converted to radiation. The major part is converted to heat, which has to be carried off by the *cooling system*. For laser up to a few kilowatts of power consumption, air-cooling, perhaps through a heat exchanger, may be sufficient. For lasers with higher consumption, however, water-cooling with up to 30 l/min at 3 bar is required.

The consumption rates for electric power and cooling water have to be borne in mind when planning or rebuilding an operating theatre for laser medicine. The floor space required can be estimated from Figures **3** and **4**.

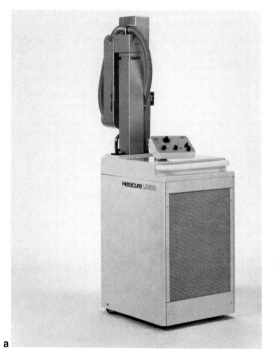
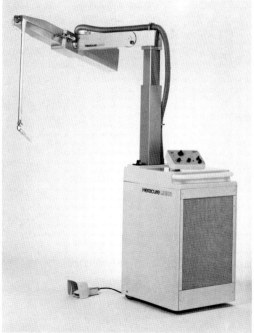

a   b

Fig. **3** CO_2 laser with articulated arm, **a** closed for transportation; **b** in working position (Photos: W. C. Heraeus GmbH, Hanau).

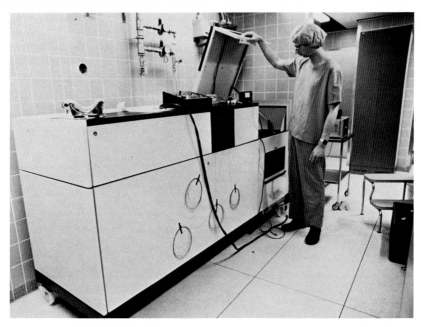

Fig. **4** Dyelaser system for PDT with integrated argon ion pumplaser; on top of the housing the remote control board. The system is operated in a seperate room and the laser radiation transmitted via a quartz fiber to the operation room (Photo: ZLL der GSF, Neuherberg/Munich).

The *light control and shutter system* regulates the laser beam parameters, power, and, in a certain range, time behavior of emission. The output power of the laser head, which is generally not equal to that at the area to be treated (see dose sensor, power meter), usually is measured by a built-in photodiode. It indicates the correct performance of the power laser and delivers the feedback signal for an output power stabilization through the power supply unit. The electrically guided mechanical shutter limits the laser emission time from cw to fractions of a second and is usually triggered by a foot switch (see later) and a timer. Sometimes two simultaneous foot switches for the surgeon and an assistant are useful to prevent an unwanted emission and increase the safety of the whole system. Additionally, an *emergency switch* is useful to prevent an unwanted emission and increase the safety of the whole system. Additionally, an *emergency switch* at the operation site has to be provided for an immediate interruption of emission by switching off the entire laser system. For a light control in the nanosecond to picosecond time domain (experimentally used for shock wave-induced lithotripsy), Q-switch or mode-lock techniques have to be applied (15) (see also chapters by Frank and by Ell et al.).

For fluorescence diagnosis of photosensitized tumors, a switching between two wavelengths of laser emission seems promising. This light control is performed by a computer-assisted adjustment of the mirrors of the laser resonator. The output power is controlled with the same computer (3).

Closely related to the light control and shutter system is the *remote control* (see Fig. **4**). Sometimes, especially to larger laser systems, such a console can be added optionally. It allows one to regulate laser parameters, which have to be adjusted with regard to the actual medical demands, from the operation site and, if necessary, under sterile conditions. The laser emission can then be individually and conveniently triggered by the foot switch, generally connected to the remote control.

Simple *radiation transfer* is the main advantage of the highly focusable laser radiation. It can be transmitted through thin flexible quartz, glass, or plastic fibers with a loss of only a few decibel per kilometer. Up to 150 W of neodymium:yttrium-aluminum-garnet (Nd:YAG) laser radiation can easily be guided by such fibers. The core diameter ranges between 50 and 1000 μm, with a total diameter of the fiber usually about twice the core, depending on the power to be transported. Most fibers are commercially available in any length. However, the application of these fibers is limited to a wavelength range of about 350 to 2500 nm. Radiation of longer wavelength can be transmitted through thallium bromide/thallium iodide (31) and chalcogenic glass fibers (13) or hollow tube wave guides (8). Since, at present, they are only of experimental value, articulated arms with internal mirror deflection have to be used (Figs. **3, 5**).

Generally, the power laser beam with an intrinsic diameter of 1 to 3 mm for most argon ion, Nd:YAG, and dye lasers up to 4 cm for a gold vapor laser has to be focused down to the fiber diameter. Misalignment produces severe losses of radiation and damage to the fiber. For practical and technical reasons, therefore, focusing is sometimes combined with *coupling* of the radiation transfer system to the laser head. Through this coupler, also gas or liquid cooling of the fiber and rinsing of the operational area can be provided.

The laser beam leaves the transmission system with a divergence similar to that through which it enters, i. e., emission cones of 8° to 15° are obtained with bare fibers. If other emission characteristics are needed, the fiber tip has to be modified by means of a *beam shaper* consisting of lenses, self-foc-integrated lenses (29), sapphire tips (9) (Fig. **6**), or fused microlenses (30). For photodynamic laser therapy in hollow organs, the emission characteristic has to be totally equalized; with a light scattering medium (36), a homogeneous integral irradiation can be obtained.

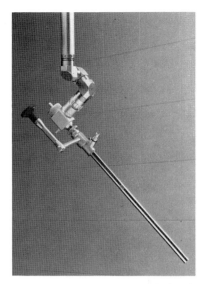

Fig. **5** Laparoscope coupled to an articulated arm for endoscopic application of middle-infrared CO_2 laser radiation (Photo: W. C. Heraeus GmbH, Hanau).

An adequate *applicator* is as important as beam shaping. For IR lasers with mirror arms, only handpieces with fixed beam shaper and deflector are possible, and rigid endoscopes of maximal about 30 cm length (Fig. **6**). Flexible fibers, however, can easily be integrated into all kinds of rigid and especially flexible endoscopes with a free channel sufficient in diameter (Fig. **7**).

By this means, laser radiation can be precisely guided to almost all sections of the gastrointestinal tract (6). For free-hand or microsurgical applications, a great variety of handpieces with and without an integrated beam shaper or binocular microscopes with attached beam guiding manipulators are available.

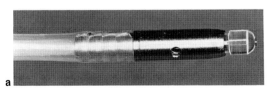
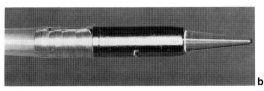

Fig. **6** Sapphire vaporization (**a**) and incision (**b**) probe connected to a quartz fiber with a metal connector. The fiber is surrounded by a cooling jacket. The coolant flows out through the borehole (Photos: ZLL der GSF, Neuherberg/Munich).

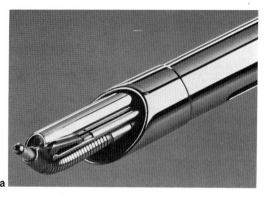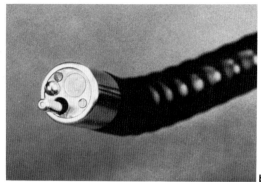

Fig. **7**   Tip of a rigid (**a**) and a flexible (**b**) endoscope with laser quartz fiber. The Albarranlever (**a**) and the flexible tip (**b**) of the instruments allow precise aiming with the laser beam under visual control (Photos: Zentralkrankenhaus der LVA, Gauting/Munich).

The most difficult problem in laser medicine is dosimetry, if one wishes to measure the amount of laser power or energy that leads to a certain laser therapeutic effect. In general, only indirect methods are available.

The simplest method is to determine, besides the time duration of laser interaction, the output power at the beam shaper or fiber tip with a *power meter*. It is assumed that no physical changes occur during the treatment. Then the characteristic values of a laser irradiation, power density (W/cm^2) and energy density (Ws/cm^2 = J/cm^2), can be calculated for the surface of the tissue and for an known geometry of irradiation.

These two values, correctly chosen, and taking into account the known time behavior of the laser radiation, and, last but not least, an experienced and skillful operator usually lead to the therapeutic effects intended.

This method fails completely, when temporary changes in the laser system itself or in the attached optical subsystems have to be taken into consideration. For example, coagula on or damage of the exit surface of the beam shaper can drastically change the emission parameters. So far, no reliable dose sensor exists, which would indicate when backscattering and reflection from humid surfaces change the dosage or when optical properties are changed by heat. Isotropic detectors, however, have been developed for the long-lasting PDT irradiation (15 to 60 minutes), which deliver a signal proportional to the varying deposition of light (26).

The maximum contribution to *safety*, when using laser medical systems, is the thorough education, training, and experience of the operator. A reliable dosimetry is an additonal prerequisite. But further equipment and installations, e. g., warning signs and interlocks, prescribed by law, technical instructions, and regulations can increase the safety for the patient, for the physician, and the assisting personnel. Eye protection with laser goggles or protection filters on eyepieces (see Fig. **1**) are a must for all persons with access to a laser area (33).

Closing Remarks

After the first 25 years of existence, the laser has proved to be a versatile and irreplacable instrument in several fields of medicine. However, it is still subject to further unforeseeable developments and is a challenge to physicians, engineers, and scientists, who all are called on to contribute to the "laser medical system" for the benefit of patient.

References

1. Bahlmann D R: The military career of the free-electron laser. Photonics Spectra 21 (4): 159–164, 1987
2. Baumgartner R, Feyh J, Götz A, Jocham D, Schneckenburger H, Stepp H, Unsöld E: Experimental study on laser-induced fluorescence of hematoporphyrin derivative (HpD) in tumor cells and animal tissue. Laser Med Surg 2:4–9, 1986

3. Baumgartner R, Lenz J, Stepp H, Unsöld E: Einrichtung zur Erzeugung verschiedener Laserwellenlängen aus demselben Lasermedium. P 37 04 388.2, Deutsches Patentamt, München 1987

4. Birngruber R: Thermal modeling in biological tissue. In: Hillenkamp F, Pratesi R, Sacchi CA (eds.): Lasers in Biology and Medicine. Plenum Press, New York 1980 (pp 77–97)

5. Brau CA: Recent developments in free-electron lasers. Laser Focus/Electro-Optics 23 (2): 40–46, 1987

6. Buess G, Unz F, Pichlmaier H: Endoskopische Techniken. Köln, Deutscher Ärzte-Verlag, 1984

7. Crystal Systems, Boston: Personal communication, 1987

8. Cunningham R: Flexible waveguide promises efficient IR delivery. Laser Appl 4 (6): 38, 1985

9. Daikuzono N, Joffe S: Artificial sapphire probe for contact photocoagulation and tissue vaporization with the Nd-YAG laser. Med Instrum 19: 173–178, 1985

10. Dickmann K: Laserdioden. Laser Magazin 2/87: 46–50, 1987

11. Dinstl K, Fischer PL: Der Laser, Grundlagen und klinische Anwendungen. Springer, Berlin 1981

12. Forrest G: Defense allocations, medical applications. Laser Focus/Electro-Optics. 22 (1): 20–28, 1986

13. Galileo Electro-Optics Corp: Personal communication, 1986

14. Harnagel G, Welch D, Cross P, Scifres D: High power laser arrays. Lasers Appl 5 (6): 135–138, 1986

15. Hofstetter A, Frank F, Keiditsch E, Wondrazek F: Intrakorporale, laserindizierte Stoßwellen-Lithotripsie (ILISL). Laser Med Surg 1: 155–158, 1985

16. Holmes L: Laser technology review. Laser Focus/Electro-Optics 23 (1): 38–48, 1987

17. Holmes L: Excimer laser. Laser Focus/Electro-Optics 22 (7): 72–81, 1986

18. Holmes L: Metal-vapor lasers: Special capabilities for special applications. Laser Focus/Electro-Optics 22 (12): 76–80, 1986

19. Holmes L: Tunable crystals and diodes lase in the infrared. Laser Focus/Electro-Optics 22 (4): 70–76, 1986

20. Holmes L: Tunable dye lasers: A versatile technology. Laser Focus/Electro-Optics 22 (2): 70–82, 1986

21. Jako GJ: Laser biomedical engineering. In: Goodman L (ed): The Biomedical Laser. Springer, Berlin 1981 (pp 175–198)

22. Jocham D, Schmiedt E, Baumgartner R, Unsöld E: Integral laser-photodynamic treatment of multifocal bladder carcinoma photosensitized by HpD. Eur Urol 12 (Suppl 1): 43–46, 1986

23. Kaplan J, Raif J: The Sharplan carbon dioxide laser in clinical surgery. In: Goldman L: The Biomedical Laser. Springer, Berlin 1981 (pp 89–97)

24. Königsmann G, Karbe E, Beck R: Application of the CO-Laser and the Ho-Laser as a surgical instrument compared with other IR-lasers and conventional instruments. Proceeding of the Symposium on Lasers in Medicine and Biology, Neuherberg, 1977. GSF-Bericht BPT 5, pp 38, 1–10, 1977

25. Lüthy W, Stalder M, Weber HP: Erbiumlaser für Mikrochirurgie. Laser Optoelektronik 19 (2): 158–159, 1987

26. Marijnissen JPA, Star WM, van Delft JL, Franken NAP: Light intensity measurement in optical phantoms and in vivo during HpD-photoradiation treatment, using a miniature light detector with isotropic response. In: Jori G, Perria C (eds): Photodynamic Therapy of Tumors and Other Diseases. Libreria Progetto Editore, Padova 1985 (pp 387–390)

27. Mathew J, Pasour JA: High gain, long-pulse free-electron laser. Postdeadline Report. Laser Focus/Electro-Optics 22 (6): 12, 1986

28. Müller G, Bader H, Greve P: 9,6 µm-CO₂-Laser für medizinische Anwendungen. Laser Med Surg 2: 86–88, 1985

29. Nippon Sheet Glass Co, Tokyo: Personal communication, 1981

30. Russo V: Fibers in medicine I. In: Ostrowsky A, Spitz B (eds): New Directions in Guided Wave and Coherent Optics, vol. I. Martinus Nijhoff, The Hague 1984

31. Sakurai Y, Nimsakul N, Tanino R, Nishimura M, Osada M: Japanese fiber-optic induced CO₂-laser in clinical application, preliminary report. In: Atsumi K, Nimsakul N (eds): Proceedings of the 4th Congress of the International Society of Laser Surgery, Tokyo 1981. Jap. Society of Laser Medicine, Tokyo 1981 (pp 1, 30–33)

32. Schneckenburger H: Time-resolved microfluorescence in biomedical diagnosis. SPIE vol. 491, High Speed Photography. Straßbourg 1984 (pp 363–366)

33. Sliney D, Wolbarsht M: Safety with lasers and other optical sources. Plenum Press, New York 1981

34. Suenaga N, Sugiyama S, Shinokura K, Atsumi K, Nimsakul N, Koyama H, Ihara A: Development of the centralized laser system. (Abstr.) Sixth Congress of the International Society of Laser Surgery and Medicine, Jerusalem 1985, 6

35. Unsöld E: Möglichkeiten und Grenzen des Lasers. Verh Dtsch Ges Inn Med, 92, 153–163, 1986

36. Unsöld E, Jocham D: Therapie photosensibilisierter Tumoren. In: Meyer HJ, Haverkampf K, Kiefhaber P (eds): Der Laser in der operativen Medizin. Edition Medizin, Weinheim 1987

37. Weber H, Herziger G: Laser, Grundlagen und Anwendungen. Physik Verlag, Weinheim 1978

Morphologic Changes with Lasers

J. Giedl

The pathologic changes of tissue caused by lasers is primarily that of thermic tissue change. There are various degrees of morphologic change up to full coagulation necrosis and tissue evaporation.

New aspects of laser use in the digestive tract, such as induction of photochemical processes in photosensitive tissue and the use of so-called athermic laser effects to produce local shock waves to break up concretions in the bile duct, do not yet have any major clinical significance and are only described marginally. Tissue changes after argon and carbon dioxide laser treatment are not discussed, since these types of laser are not relevant for laser endoscopy in the gastrointestinal tract today.

The degree and extent of the morphologic changes caused by laser treatment depend on the physical parameters of the laser beam (power, density, beam diameter, laser wavelength, and pulse duration of therapy) and the optic and thermic properties of the tissue treated (see p. 3–10).

Thermal Effects in Liver-Tissue

The main morphologic changes after laser therapy are described with the neodymium: yttrium-aluminum-garnet (Nd:YAG) laser 1064 nm in prolonged application and with cw noncontact technique.

The light energy absorbed by the tissue after Nd:YAG laser therapy is directly changed to heat and induces warming of the tissue. If the energy absorbed is low, heat can be conducted away without tissue damage taking place. If the absorbed energy crosses a threshold value, there is an increase in temperature that leads to coagulation necrosis owing to protein being denatured. If the temperature in the tissue exceeds 100°, the water-containing tissue in the center of the beam evaporates.

Changes in Morphology

The acute changes in morphology after Nd:YAG laser treatment in vivo are shown in the liver (Figs. 1, 2).

Central cavity development owing to evaporation.

Thin carbonization zone composed of formless eosinophil proteins and carbonized material (less than 0.1 mm).

Layer of peripheral cavity development (0.2 to 0.5 mm) with cavities of various sizes that are produced by cell water evaporation and are characterized by bunched groups of cells with densely coagulated cytoplasma and nuclei.

Acidophilic zone (1.5 to 4.5 mm) composed of even striations and cells with eosinophilic cytoplasm and pyknotic nuclei.

Transitional zone. Hepatocytes with more than normally acidophilic cytoplasm, but with basophilic coloration of the endoplasmic reticulum, which is absent in acidophilic zone.

Hyperemic zone. Marked hyperemia is in the sinusoids. There is much dissociation of the liver cells in this layer.

In fresh, dead liver tissue the hyperemic zone is absent after Nd:YAG laser therapy. The same sort of changes are found in the gastrointestinal organs that are accessible to endoscopy, such as the esophagus, stomach, and colon.

Acute Lesions

At 30 J/cm^2, marked mucosal edema is found in the treated area after laser therapy. There is also shedding of the surface epithelium and dissociation of the epithelial cells.

At energies up to 100 J/cm^2, coagulation necrosis takes place into the submucosa or as far as the muscle layer (Fig. 3). The collagen fibers in the edematous submucosa appear shrunken and significantly thickened. They are

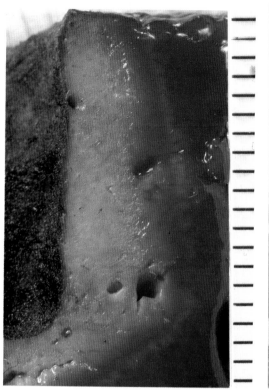

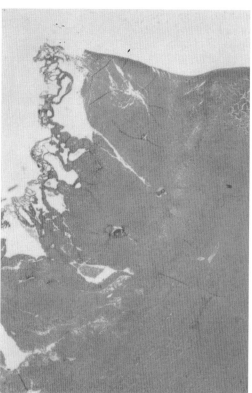

Fig. 1 Macroscopically visible layers in Nd:YAG laser lesions in liver tissue in vivo (wavelength 1064 nm, noncontact, distance 5 mm, 60 W, 3 s). Central cavity in the left of the picture with blackish carbonization zone. The broad, yellowish zone is the coagulation zone. The narrow yellowish zone on the right is the hyperthermic zone.

Fig. 2 Histologic cross-section of an in vivo lesion of the liver due to Nd:YAG laser (wavelength 1320 nm, noncontact, distance 5 mm, 24 W, 3 s). From left to right, central cavity, narrow carbonization zone, peripheral cavity development, broad coagulation zone, broad hyperemic zone, (H & E; × 20).

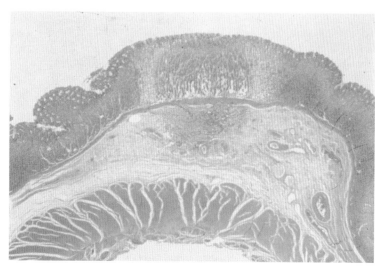

Fig. 3 Nd:YAG laser (1064 nm, noncontact, distance 5 mm, 80 W, 3 s). Dog stomach; acute lesion in vivo. In the middle, coagulation necrosis can be seen reaching into the submucosa. The propria, mucous membrane, and submucosa at the sides of the lesion are intact (H & E; × 5).

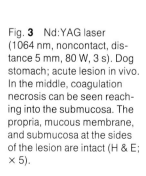

arched or angular in form and under high magnification (×400) show marked cross-striation (7).

Initially (30 minutes after exposure), the submucosal vessels are open, with no thrombi, and their walls appear to be intact. After only 4 hours, there are many thrombosed capillaries, bleeding, and individual leukocyte infiltration.

Apart from a minimal edema, there are no unusual findings at this time in the smooth muscle. One day after laser therapy, the edema in the laser zone area has regressed. The treated area stands out from its still edematous surroundings. An extensive mucosal ulceration develops, reaching into the submucosa. Thrombocytes are found in the capillaries and there are thromboses in the venules. The arterioles show fibrinoid necrosis of their walls. The muscle fiber necroses are now clearly visible. The non-nucleated muscle fibers are condensed to a compact hyalin mass, and homogeneous band-shaped coagulation necrosis is present.

Chronic Changes

From 4 to 14 Days

After a few days, depending on the physical parameters (see above), the superficial and deep tissue changes with the Nd:YAG laser are significantly more extensive than those in the acute phase. This is irreversible because all damage is already achieved at 58°C, although then is no immediate macro- or microscopic evidence of this. The increase in necrosis is promoted by multiple distribution of the Nd:YAG in tissue and by heat conduction. On the other hand, the higher thrombosis potential and the consequent blood perfusion disturbance can play a role in the increased ulceration. For the endoscopist, this means that he must expect larger superficial and deep lesions than the acute lesions visible at endoscopy, and that the full extent of the lesions can only be recognized after a few days.

After 3 to 4 days, repair and resorption processes can be recognized, coming in from the surrounding vital areas.

On the surface reepithelialization is seen, with a single epithelial layer originating in the bordering intact mucosa, and growing out to cover the necrotic tissue. Organization of the laser necrosis takes place through granulation tissue growing in from the submucosa. Ingrowing capillaries, fibroblast proliferation, and phagocytes dominate the picture in laser necrosis. Renewal formation of smooth muscle cells takes place, mainly from migratory transformed fibroblasts of the granulation tissue (7).

After About 5 Weeks

At this point, the ulceration is more or less healed. The mucosa looks normal histologically and with the naked eye, although a relatively small connective tissue scar can be seen in the submucosa and the muscularis propria (5).

New Developments

Contact Laser Therapy

The tissue lesion produced by contact laser therapy (sapphire tip or metal tip, the "hot

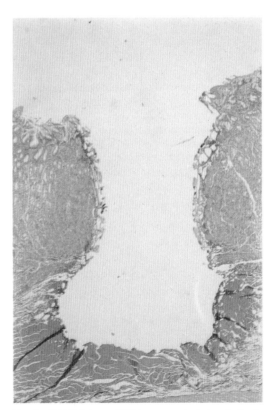

Fig. 4   Nd:YAG laser (1064 nm, contact, hemispherical sapphire contact tip, SLT, Japan; 18 W, 3 s) Dog stomach; acute lesion in vivo. Punctate central cavity reaching deep into the submucosa and extending there. Coagulation necrosis at the edges (H & E; × 40).

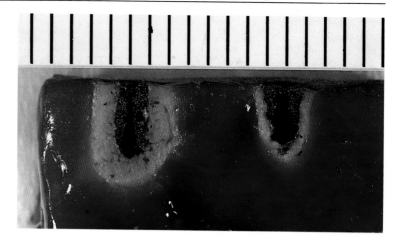

Fig. **5** Comparison of the lesions produced with the Nd:YAG laser of 1064 nm wavelength on the right and of 1320 nm on the left (in vitro, noncontact, distance 5 mm, 60 and 24 W, 3 s).

tip") depends on the laser power applied and the total energy, as well as on the pressure exerted by the tip on the tissue surface. Visible morphologic changes include:

- The central vaporization defect shows the shape of the contact tip (punch defect) (Fig. **4**).
- Irregular vaporization defect boundaries owing to adhesion of tissue to the contact tip and coagulated tissue tearing loose when the tip is removed.
- The coagulation zone in the submucosa is significantly broader with the contact method than with the noncontact method; in the mucosa it is not so broad. These effects can be seen with the 1,064 nm as well as with the 1,318 nm Nd:YAG laser.
- The thermic edema caused by the laser is significantly less with the contact method than with the noncontact method (1).

Overall, the acute visible morphologic tissue changes correspond generally to the lesions visible after a few days.

Nd:YAG different wave lengths

Comparing lesions of similar size, and therefore similar amount of denatured tissue, with a wavelength of 1,320 nm in prolonged use, in contrast to the laser with a 1064 nm wavelength, the 1,320 nm wavelength Nd:YAG laser shows:

- Less vaporization (narrower central cavity)
- A smaller carbonization zone

- Significant decrease in peripheral cavity development
- A broad coagulation zone (Fig. **5**).

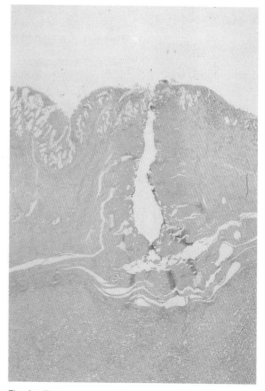

Fig. **6** Flash lamp pulsed Nd:YAG impulse laser. Bile duct wall of the dog in vivo. Coagulation necrosis with thin, central cavity development. Impulse duration 2 ms. Impulse energy 2 J. Total impulse energy 16 J (H & E; × 40).

Pulsed Nd:YAG lasers

In flash pulsation Nd:YAG laser (2 ms, 2 Ip.p. 4 Hz, 1s) used for laser lithotripsy of biliary calculi, there is a narrow, punctate, cavity development, surrounded by a narrow coagulation necrosis (Fig. **6**). With the Q-switched Nd:YAG laser light, energy is altered to pure mechanical energy. Ultrashort shock waves are developed (2, 3, 6). The morphologically visible tissue changes caused by this are not thermic; they are mechanical damage. Depending on the number of shock waves and the duration of therapy, there is mechanical tearing of the tissues with possible hematoma development (3, 6) (Fig. **7**).

Laser Therapy of Photosensitized Tissue

Systematically given photosensitizers (hematoporphyrin derivatives, Photophrin II, etc.) with high affinity for (pre)malignant changes induce intracellular photochemical processes at irradiation with light of a certain wavelength (e. g., 630 nm), and this leads to cell death. The histologic picture is coagulation necrosis (Fig. **8**).

The aim is to treat precursors or early forms of malignant tumors (adenoma, early carcinoma) in the gastrointestinal tract (4).

With this type of treatment, attention must be paid to the unsolved problem of exact histologic confirmation of the diagnosis, the exact depth of the tumor, and the precise clinical exclusion of lymph node metastases. Future aspects of this therapy include the development of more effective photosensitizers and the combination of photodynamic therapy with other therapeutic modalities, such as radiotherapy and hyperthermia.

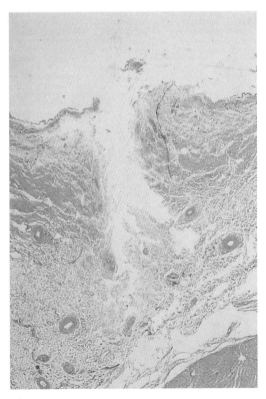

Fig. 7   Q-switched Nd:YAG laser. Bile duct wall in beef liver. Mechanical destruction of the epithelium and the duct wall after 1500 pulses (8 ns, 30 mJ, 20 Hz). Duration of therapy 150 s (H & E; × 40).

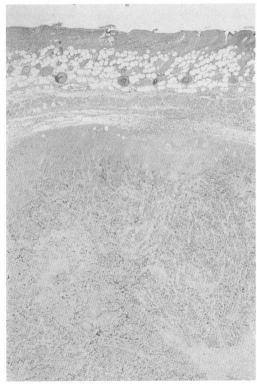

Fig. 8   Coagulation necrosis of a human colon carcinoma transplanted on a nude mouse after systematic photosensitizers and laser therapy at 75 J/cm². The mouse skin is at the top (H & E; × 40).

References

1. Ell Ch, Hochberger J, Lux G: Clinical experience of non-contact and contact Nd-YAG laser therapy for inoperable malignant stenoses of the oesophagus and stomach. Lasers Med Sci 1: 143–146, 1986
2. Ell Ch, Hochberger J, Müller D, Zirngibl H, Giedl J, Lux G, Demling L: Laser lithotripsy of gallstone by means of a pulsed neodymium-YAG laser – in vitro and animal experiments. Endoscopy 18: 92–94, 1986
3. Ell Ch, Wondrazek F, Frank F, Hochberger J, Lux G, Demling L: Laser induced shockwave lithotripsy of gallstones (LISL). Endoscopy 18: 95–96, 1986
4. Kato H, Kawaguchi M, Konaka C, Nishimiya K, Kawate N, Yoneyama K, Kinoshita K, Noguchi M, Ishii M, Shirai M, Hirano T, Aizawa K, Hayata Y: Evaluation of photodynamic therapy in gastric cancer. Lasers Med Sci 1: 67–74, 1986
5. Kelly DF, Bown SG, Calder BM, Pearson H, Weaver BMQ, Swain CP, Salmon PR: Histological changes following ND YAG laser photocoagulation of canine gastric mucosa. Gut 24: 914–920, 1983
6. Schmeller NT, Hofstetter AG, Pensel J, Thomas S, Frank F, Wondrazek F: Laserinduzierte Stoßwellen-lithotripsie (LISL). Laser Med Surg 3: 184–193, 1987
7. Zimmermann I, Stern J, Keiditsch E, Frank F, Hofstetter A: Restitution und Reparation nach ausgedehnter primärer und sekundärer Neodym-YAG-Lasernekrose der Rattenharnblase. Laser Med Surg 3: 215–223, 1987

Upper Gastrointestinal Tract

Hemostasis

P. Rutgeerts and G. Vantrappen

Upper gastrointestinal bleeding still has an overall mortality of about 10%. The incidence of this often dramatic emergency is estimated at 1 in 1000 per year. Prognostic factors for outcome have now clearly been defined (1, 2, 32, 34). About 70 to 80% of the patients have already stopped bleeding when admitted to the hospital. No transfusion or only a few units are required. Endoscopy in these patients visualizes a nonbleeding lesion, mostly without stigmata of recent hemorrhage (SRH). The evolution will be uneventful and any aggressive therapy may harm the patient. Twenty to 30% of the patients are admitted with arterial hypotension and continue to bleed or rebleed while in the hospital. These patients have high transfusion requirements and are at high risk.

Severe bleeding almost always originates from peptic ulcers or from esophageal or fundic varices. In patients with severe bleeding an upper gastrointestinal endoscopy should be performed as soon as possible after resuscitation. There is no doubt that the diagnostic yield of early endoscopy in upper gastrointestinal hemorrhage is superior of that of a barium swallow.

The timing of endoscopy influences the frequency of active bleeding present at endoscopy (34). If performed within 12 hours of admission, 41% of the patients have active bleeding. When endoscopy is performed more than 12 hours after admission, the incidence of active bleeding is about 30%. In a survey by the American Society for Gastrointestinal Endoscopy (34) actived bleeding at endoscopy was associated with a mortality rate of 16.1%; if there was no active bleeding, the mortality declined to 6.7%. The nature of the bleeding lesion has prognostic importance. Therapeutic efforts should be directed to those patients who continue to bleed or are likely to rebleed. It is critical to identify these high-risk groups.

Bleeding from esophagitis, Mallory-Weiss tears, neoplasms, gastric erosions, erosive duodenitis, and vascular malformations is usually mild. When peptic ulcers or varices are diagnosed at endoscopy, the finding of SRH predicts further bleeding.

In 1978 Foster et al. (10) identified three endoscopic SRH as predictors of continuing or recurrent bleeding: fresh bleeding from the lesion, fresh or altered clot or black slough adherent to the lesion, and a vessel protruding from the base or the margin of an ulcer. Griffiths et al. (14) confirmed the prognostic importance of the visible vessel. Accurate prospective data were obtained by Storey et al. (36) and Swain et al. (38). It is easy to identify a spurting hemorrhage or a pulsating pseudoaneurysm as arterial in origin. Identification of a nonbleeding artery is more subjective. According to Storey et al. (36) and Swain et al. (38) a nonbleeding artery appears on endoscopy as an elevated red or blue spot, resistant to gentle washing, often associated with a red clot and almost always solitary in the ulcer crater. Overall recurrent bleeding occurred in 85% of ulcers presenting with spurting hemorrhage at endoscopy, in 51% of ulcers with a nonbleeding visible vessel, in 5% of ulcers with other SRH, and in 0% of ulcers without stigmata.

These data were challenged recently by Wara (39), who found a lower rebleeding rate

(32%) of ulcers with nonbleeding visible vessels. He suggested that a visible vessel carries a high rebleeding risk only when oozing hemorrhage or an overlying clot is present at endoscopy.

Another recent study by Bornman et al. (4) showed that the association of shock with important endoscopic signs is a stronger predictor of rebleeding than either shock or important signs alone.

The diagnosis of bleeding from varices (3) is definite if a varix is seen to be spurting or oozing blood. The presence of a clot, an erosion, or an ecchymosis suggests bleeding from varices. A recently described SRH from varices was a white "nipple," protruding from the varix, which was probably a fibrin plug (6). When the source of bleeding in a cirrhotic patient with varices cannot be ascertained, endoscopy should be repeated when bleeding recurs to determine the variceal or nonvariceal origin of the bleeding.

One decade ago patients with severe upper gastrointestinal hemorrhage were candidates for emergency surgery, carrying a mortality of approximately 25% in contrast with the 3% mortality of elective surgery for upper gastrointestinal hemorrhage.

Several methods of hemostasis in upper gastrointestinal bleeding have been developed and were evaluated in animal experiments, human pilot studies, controlled clinical trials, and randomized comparative studies.

The ultimate benefit of endoscopic hemostasis for the patient with upper gastrointestinal hemorrhage is reduction of mortality, but benefit might also encompass lowered morbidity rates and reduced cost of patient care.

Efficient endoscopic hemostasis would reduce mortality due to bleeding; by avoiding emergency surgery, it would also decrease the often lethal postoperative complications.

This chapter deals with the use of the neodymium:yttrium-aluminum-garnet (Nd:YAG) laser in the treatment of bleeding ulcers and visible vessels. YAG laser photocoagulation of bleeding esophageal varices will be briefly discussed. Based on our experience and on data from the literature, we shall try to define the current place of the YAG laser in the treatment of upper gastrointestinal bleeding.

Patients

From 1978 untill December 1986, we treated 344 patients with laser for acute upper gastrointestinal hemorrhage. In our pilot studies all lesions were treated, not only ulcers, but also gastric and duodenal erosions, Mallory-Weiss tears, and varices. When it became clear from our data and from the literature that these lesions often stop bleeding spontaneously, therapy was only directed to bleeding ulcers with vessels. For bleeding varices, other, better therapy modalities became available.

In total, 275 patients with bleeding ulcers were treated by YAG laser photocoagulation. The age distribution of these patients is shown in Figure 1. Fifty-five percent of patients with ulcers were over the age 60 years, and 35% had one or more underlying severe medical problems. Only 30% of the patients had a history of peptic ulcer disease, and 41% of the patients had taken nonsteroidal anti-inflammatory drugs.

All patients were treated in the endoscopy department after resuscitation in the emergence department or intensive care units. Endoscopy was almost always performed within 12 hours of admission. When we started to use YAG laser treatment in patients with very severe bleeding, it was performed under general anesthesia and intubation. Now, general anesthesia is only rarely used. When careful inspection of the upper gastrointestinal tract is not possible due to the large amount of blood present, the stomach is cleansed with ice-cold saline through a large gastric tube. Severe bleeders are carefully monitored throughout

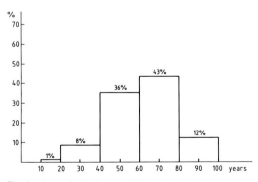

Fig. 1   Age distribution of 275 patients with bleeding from peptic ulcers treated by Nd:YAG laser photocoagulation.

the procedure and thereafter. Coagulation disorders are corrected and blood transfusion, parenteral alimentation, and H_2-blocking agents are administered intravenously.

Methods

Nd:YAG Laser Photocoagulation

The modalities of power and exposure setting for YAG photocoagulation and the mechanisms of hemostasis have been studied experimentally in dogs (5, 11, 28). Hemostasis is achieved by protein coagulation, denaturation of collagen, formation of platelet thrombi, and vessel constriction. These features occur at tissue temperatures between 60° and 80°C. A temperature plateau of ± 70°C at the tissue level is best achieved by repeated short (0.5 to 1 s) pulses of high power (70 to 90 W). At higher temperatures, such as 100°C, vaporization occurs and an ulcer is created. When hemostasis is attempted, this is dangerous for two reasons: Ulcer formation increases the risk of transmural injury and perforation, and the cutting effect of the laser may incise the vessel and cause severe bleeding.

In the clinical setting most gastroenterologists use high-power and short pulses, although some (31) prefer continuous photocoagulation. When severe bleeding is present, it may be necessary to use longer exposure times because some energy is carried away by blood flow. The working distance varies between 0.5 and 1.5 cm. It is sometimes necessary to treat a lesion at very short distances, e. g., when treatment is performed in a deformed bulb; other lesions, such as those in the fundic area, may have to be treated at greater distances. Power setting and pulse duration have, then, to be changed accordingly. The output of the laser beam at the fiber tip should be checked regularly. Visible tissue erosion should always be avoided. Most endoscopists now use the flexible transmission fiber with carbon dioxide gas. Kiefhaber still uses the triconical quartz fiber built in the scope.

The flexible fiber should be cleaned after each series of pulses in order to remove coagulated blood, so that the desired output is obtained. High-rate gas flow can be very useful when treating an artery spurting blood but should not be used when treating an oozing or nonbleeding vessel. Accidents have occured due to overdistension, e. g., perforation of tear

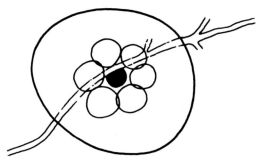

Fig. 2 Nd:YAG laser photocoagulation, when directly applied to a nonbleeding visible vessel, may induce torrential hemorrhage. Therefore photocoagulation is first carried out around the vessel and therapy is completed by photocoagulation of the vessel itself.

rupture provoked by belching. A minimal gas flow (5 ml/s), however, is necessary to prevent plugging of the tip, resulting in fiber burn. Cleansing of the fiber tip with water avoids distension problems, but the water jet may prevent correct aiming of the pilot laser. When treating a visible vessel with YAG laser alone, photocoagulation should be started circumferentially to the vessel (Fig. 2), followed by photocoagulation of the vessel itself. At the end of the session, the vessel or "sentinel clot" should always be completely destroyed, leaving a flat lesion (Fig. 3) in order to assure complete closure of the vessel. Direct application of high energy to the vessel may induce dramatic hemorrhage, especially when a branch of the gastroduodenal artery is involved.

Combined Injection Therapy and YAG Photocoagulation

The success rate of YAG laser hemostasis in patients with severe bleeding from visible vessels in ulcers was disappointing in our hands. Although an initial hemostasis rate of more than 80% was obtained, recurrence of bleeding occured frequently, and up to 50% of these patients had to undergo surgery. Therefore, we tried to improve the success rate of YAG laser therapy in two ways. The first method was based on the combination of local epinephrine injection (to stop or decrease the bleeding at least temporarily) followed by YAG laser photocoagulation (to obliterate and destroy completely the vessel that caused the

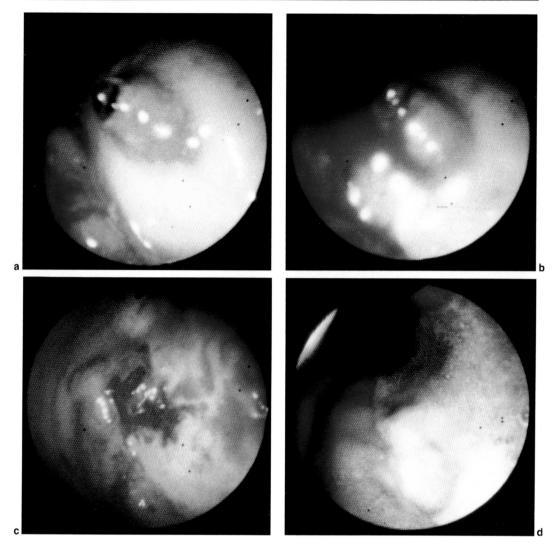

Fig. 3 **a** A large ulcer with central nonbleeding visible vessel, presenting as a pseudoaneurysm. **b** Oozing from the vessel occurs when Nd:YAG laser therapy is started **c** Further photocoagulation controls hemorrhage and is continued until the vessel is completely flat **d** The ulcer heals quickly in the following weeks.

bleeding (26). For small ulcers, 2 ml of an epinephrine solution 1:10,000 was injected through a sclerotherapy needle submucosally in each quadrant of the ulcer rim (Fig. **4**). For large ulcers with central vessel, the solution was injected in the ulcer base around the vessel. After injection, the lesion was treated by Nd:YAG laser photocoagulation. When bleeding was not controlled by laser, a second injection was given to arrest or slow down the bleeding in order to facilitate further YAG laser therapy.

The second method of treatment consisted of repeated therapy sessions. In the early years of laser therapy this was only rarely done because of the penetration depth of the laser and the fear of perforation.

Results

In the pilot studies YAG laser photocoagulation resulted in an initial hemostasis rate of 95%; rebleeding occured in 22% of cases.

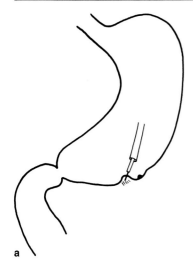

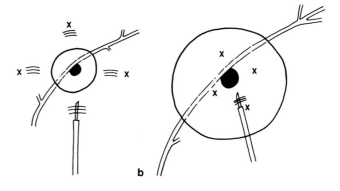

Fig. 4 **a** Submucosal injection of 2 ml of epinephrine 1 % is carried out at the edge of the ulcer in each quadrant. **b** When the ulcer is large the injection is not carried out at the edge but directly into the ulcer base around the protruding vessel.

When we compared retrospectively overall data with results obtained in ulcers with visible vessels, it appeared that the definitive hemostasis rate was much lower in this subgroup of patients (29) (Table **1**).

Subsequently, we undertook a *randomized controlled trial of YAG laser photocoagulation* in upper gastrointestinal hemorrhage. For ethical reasons, patients with spurting hemorrhage were not randomized but were always treated by laser. Spurting arterial bleeding could be controlled in 87% of the patients (20 of 23 patients), but the recurrence rate of bleeding was high (55%). The incidence of surgery was less in this group (61%) compared with an historical control group (95%). Patients with active oozing hemorrhage and patients with fresh SRH, i. e., with fresh clot or a

Table **1** Comparison of Overall Results of YAG Laser Therapy with Results in Ulcers with Visible Vessels

	Overall Data (All Lesions)	Ulcers with Vessels
Number	130	36
Initial hemostasis	124 (95%)	30 (83%)
Rebleeding	29 (22%)	18 (50%)
Surgery	20 (15%)	18 (50%)
Mortality	22 (17%)	11 (31%)

visible vessel, were included in the controlled randomized trial. Details of this study have been published elsewhere (27) but can be summarized as follows (Table **2**).

Table **2** Controlled Data on YAG Laser Therapy of Active Nonspurting Bleeding and Fresh Stigmata of Bleeding

	Overall		Ulcers with Severe Bleeding (Transfusion > 5 U)	
	Laser	Control	Laser	Control
No. patients	63	66	30	27
No hemostasis	6 (10%)	21 (32%) p = 0.0038	4 (13%)	14 (52%) p = 0.0045
Operation rate	3 (5%)	11 (17%) p = 0.059	3 (10%)	10 (37%) p = 0.035
Mortality rate	8 (13%)	10 (15%)	7 (23%)	7 (26%)

Table **3** Retrospective Comparison of Results of Combined Epinephrine 1 : 10,000 Injection and YAG Laser and Repeated Therapy with Results of One Therapy Session of YAG Alone in Treatment of Visible Vessels (Bleeding and Nonbleeding)

	Laser Therapy Alone (One Session)	Epinephrine Injection + Laser (Repeated Therapy)
No. of patients	134	141
Initial hemostasis	114 (85%)	137 (97%)
Definitive hemostasis		
after one session	81 (62%)	101 (71%)
after repeated therapy	–	125 (89%)
Emergency surgery	40 (30%)	15 (11%)
Mortality during hospital stay	28 (21%)	10 (8%)

Overall, YAG laser photocoagulation significantly reduced the duration of bleeding, the recurrence rate, and the need for emergency operation. The benefit of YAG laser therapy was even more striking in the subgroup of patients with severely bleeding peptic ulcers (i. e., transfusion requirements of more than 5 U).

To improve the results of YAG laser therapy, we *combined YAG photocoagulation with injection of a solution of epinephrine 1 : 10,000.* This combined treatment was compared with the results of YAG laser therapy alone. The results are summarized in Table **3**.

Since the comparative study was not carried out in a randomized fashion, statistical significance was not calculated. It is obvious, however, that the results of combined therapy were much better than those of YAG laser therapy alone.

Importance of Repeated Therapy for Hemostasis

The results of combined epinephrine and laser therapy for bleeding from ulcers with visible vessels was analyzed in order to determine prognostically important factors. The specific aim was to identify those patients in whom a second photocoagulation should be attempted and those in whom repeated endoscopic hemostasis could increase the risk by postponing inevitable emergency surgery. The initial

hemostasis rate was 97% (137 of 141 patients). Definitve hemostasis was obtained after one therapy session in 72% (101 patients), whereas definitve hemostasis was achieved with repeated endoscopic therapy in 89% (125 patients). Negative predictive factors for outcome after endoscopic therapy were ulcer size greater than 2 cm in diameter, ulcers located on the posterior wall of the bulb or in the postbulbar region.

Complications

Perforation with free abdominal gas occurred in 2 of 344 patients (0.6%). The most common complication was aspiration pneumonia, which occured in about 10% of the patients with severe bleeding. The exact incidence is difficult to assess. Although this complication is seen after diagnostic endoscopy in the patient with upper gastrointestinal bleeding, the risk of aspiration is probably increased when the duration of the procedure is increased due to endoscopic hemostasis. Laser-induced massive hemorrhage was rare and could be controlled by continuing therapy. Damage to the endoscope by laser carried a high cost. The frequency of fiber burn depends on the gas flow used. Cut and polish of the fiber had to be performed routinely.

Discussion

The therapeutic applications of fiberoptic endoscopy in the field of gastroenterology are rapidly expanding. Of the various therapeutic applications to date, a major focus has been on the treatment of gastrointestinal bleeding. Laser photocoagulation has been one of the most exciting endoscopic approaches for treatment of various bleeding lesions.

The controversy that existed as to which of the gastrointestinal lasers, the argon or the Nd:YAG laser, should be used has been solved by clinical use. The 1.06 µm YAG laser is preferred because its beam is not absorbed by overlying blood and because its greater depth of penetration makes this laser more efficacious than the argon laser in treating large bleeding vessels. The fear of excessive transmural injury by the YAG laser beam causing gut perforation proved to be unwarranted and this laser was quite safe in the clinical setting.

After the pioneering work of P. Kiefhaber (20) in Germany and R. Dwyer in the United

States (7) a number of centers gained extensive experience with YAG laser hemostasis of gastrointestinal bleeding lesions. Kiefhaber (19) reported on successful results in 94% of 692 unselected patients with various causes of upper gastrointestinal bleeding. Sander et al. (31) and Shönekäs (33) also reported very good results with Nd:YAG laser photocoagulation in a large series of patients with gastrointestinal bleeding. However, as shown by our pilot studies, overall results have to be interpreted with care, since these tend to overestimate the efficacy of the technique because a number of lesions treated, e. g., erosions, Mallory-Weiss tears, tumors, and postpolypectomy hemorrhages, have low bleeding potential and mostly stop bleeding spontaneously. In severe bleeding from ulcers with visible vessels, initial hemostasis is readily achieved but recurrent bleeding occurs frequently. Therefore, the true benefit of endoscopic hemostasis can only be determined by randomized controlled studies. These studies are, however, difficult to carry out for ethical reasons. In our own studies, therefore, we did not include patients with severe bleeding and those with spurting vessels. These were always treated by laser.

Three of six controlled trials (8, 16, 21, 23, 27, 37) using Nd:YAG laser photocoagulation for hemostasis showed significant benefit. The trial of McLeod et al. (23) showed significant reduction of rebleeding and emergency surgery in patients with severe bleeding. Our trial also showed significant reduction of rebleeding and emergency surgery rate when actively bleeding ulcers and ulcers with SRH were combined (27). The recent trial of Swain et al. (37) showed, besides significant reduction of rebleeding and emergency surgery rate, also a significant reduction of mortality.

The negative trials have some methodologic drawbacks. In the trial of Ihre et al. (16) only a very small number of patients were included. Escourrou et al. (8) included in their series endoscopic failures, i. e., patients in whom the lesions could not be reached by the endoscope. Krejs et al. (21) excluded patients with severe bleeding from the trial.

To increase the success rate of endoscopic YAG laser therapy, epinephrine 1‰ injection may be of value with YAG laser therapy. Also, repeated therapy for recurring bleeding may increase the success rate in selected patients, i. e., in patients with small ulcers and ulcers that do not erode large caliber serosal vessels, e. g., the gastroduodenal artery. In our studies repeated therapy was successful in 80% of the patients with recurrence after a first therapy session.

The efficacy of Nd:YAG laser photocoagulation for hemostasis is now well established. A major disadvantage is the cost of the laser, particularly if it is only used for hemostasis. Fortunately, laser photocoagulation has other fields of application, such as palliative therapy of esophageal and colorectal carcinomas and therapy of angiodysplasia.

Other and cheaper methods of endoscopic hemostasis have been developed. Monopolar electrocoagulation is probably effective but carries a high perforation risk. Multipolar electrocoagulation (Bicap)carries a lesser risk, but its efficacy remains to be determined. Although the experimental and pilot data on bipolar electrocoagulation are encouraging, only a few controlled trials have been carried out thus far. Two controlled trials (13, 18) showed no benefit for multipolar electrocoagulation using the 7 Fr (2.3 mm) Bicap probe. A recent controlled trial by Laine (22) showed a significant reduction in continued bleeding, transfusion requirements, hospital stay, and mortality for patients treated with Bicap electrocoagulation. In this study the 10 Fr Bicap was used (3.2 mm).

Comparative experimental studies of YAG laser and Bicap suggest that both modalities are equally effective. In a small randomized clinical trial by Goff (12), Bicap seemed somewhat more efficacious than YAG laser (no rebleeding in three of eight patients after YAG, 6 of 11 after Bicap; p <0.1). In that study the results of either therapy were poor.

In a large randomized comparison carried out in our department (30), we showed that in patients presenting at endoscopy with peptic ulcer and a spurting or oozing vessel or with a nonbleeding visible vessel, YAG laser and Bicap were equally effective and resulted in definitive hemostasis in about 72% after one treatment and 86 to 88% after two treatment sessions. It should be stressed that in the latter study we always used pretreatment with epinephrine 1 : 10,000 injection in both groups. The Bicap probe diameter (10 Fr versus 7 Fr) seems to be very important for the efficacy of multipolar electrocoagulation of bleeding ulcers. Consequently, the application of Bicap always nessesitates the use of large channel endoscopes, whereas the laser fiber can be introduced through the channel of each standard gastroscope. The output of the Bicap unit seems less critical. We obtained very good results with the 25 W Bicap unit at output 10. With the 50 W Bicap unit, 5 is the output to be used.

Another thermal modality, the heater probe, has been studied experimentally and seems to be very effective for hemostasis. Broad clinical data, however, are lacking. Johnston et al. (17) compared the heater probe in a nonrandomized study with the YAG laser and found the heater probe to be more effective than the YAG laser. Nonrandomized comparisons, however, need to be interpreted with care.

A very attractive alternative for endoscopic hemostasis of upper gastrointestinal bleeding is sclerotherapy. This technique, frequently used for variceal bleeding, was introduced for hemostasis by Soehendra (35). He reported on very good results of injection with epinephrine 1 : 10,000 and polidocanol 1% in nonselected cases of gastrointestinal hemorrhage. A number of Japanese endoscopists use injections of absolute alcohol and epinephrine solutions (15) for hemostasis and obtained high success rates.

On the basis of experimental and clinical studies, we used to believe that injection should be combined with thermal methods to achieve optimal efficacy (25). Preliminary results of a randomized comparison, however, show that injection with epinephrine 1% followed by injection with 3 to 5 ml polidocanol 1% may be as efficacious as injection with epinephrine 1‰ followed by YAG laser (24).

Acute variceal bleeding can be controlled by Nd:YAG laserphotocoagulation, and high success rates for laser hemostasis of bleeding varices have been published. However, most investigators agree that the recurrence rate of bleeding is very high. This was clearly demonstrated by Fleischer (9) in a controlled trial of YAG laser photocoagulation for hemostasis of bleeding esophageal varices. In this study initial hemostasis was achieved in seven of ten patients with bleeding varices treated by laser, compared with none of ten control subjects. However, in three of seven patients in the laser group bleeding recurred. There were no differences in transfusion requirements between treated and control patients. Endoscopic hemostasis of bleeding esophageal varices can be achieved by sclerotherapy, and by repeated sclerotherapy sessions, eradication of esophageal varices can be obtained, decreasing the risk for rebleeding. Therefore, this modality is now the therapy of choice for bleeding from esophageal varices.

Summary

Nd:YAG laser photocoagulation is a very effective treatment modality for acute upper gastrointestinal hemorrhage. Endoscopic therapy of severe bleeding is very demanding and much skill is necessary to expose the bleeding site and to coagulate the lesion. The laser can be used safely, and effective treatment lowers emergency surgery rates. Mortality rates are less influenced by successful hemostasis because most deaths from patients with upper gastrointestinal bleeding are due to underlying disease.

Other therapy modalities, e. g., bipolar electrocoagulation, and injection methods, have been proposed. We are convinced that the combined use of injection therapy and YAG laser obtains optimal results.

References

1. Allan R, Dykes P: A study of the factors influencing mortality rates from gastrointestinal hemorrhage. Q J Med (NS) 45: 533–538, 1976
2. Avery-Jones F: Hematemesis and melaena with special reference to causation and to factors influencing the mortality from bleeding peptic ulcers. Gastroenterology 30: 166–169, 1956
3. Beppu K, Inokuchi K, Koyanagi N: Prediction of variceal hemorrhage by esophageal endoscopy. Gastrointest Endosc 27: 213–218, 1981
4. Bornman PC, Theodorou NA, Shuttleworth RD, Essel HP, Marks IN: Importance of hypovolemic shock and endoscopic signs in predicting recurrent hemorrhage from peptic ulceration: A prospective evaluation. Br Med J 291: 245–247, 1985
5. Bown SG, Salmon PR, Storey DW: Neodymium-YAG laser photocoagulation in the dog stomach. Gut 21: 818–825, 1980
6. Chung RS, Lewis JW: The platelet-fibrin plug in esophageal variceal hemorrhage: The mount St. Helens' sign. (Letter.) Gastrointest Endosc 30: 270, 1984

7. Dwyer RM, Yellin AE, Craig J: Gastric hemostasis by laser phototherapy in man. JAMA 236: 1383–1386, 1976

8. Escourrou J, Frexinos J, Bommelaer G, et al: Prospective randomized study of YAG photocoagulation in gastrointestinal bleeding. In: Atsumi, Nimsakul N (eds): Proceedings of Laser. Tokyo 1981 (pp. 5–30)

9. Fleischer D:Endoscopic Nd:YAG laser therapy for active esophageal variceal bleeding. Gastrointest, Endosc 31: 4–9, 1985

10. Foster DN, Miloszewski KJA, Losowsky MS: Stigmata of recent haemorrhage in diagnosis and prognosis of upper gastrointestinal bleeding. Br Med J 1: 11763–1177, 1978

11. Geboes K, Rutgeerts P, Vantrappen G: A microscopic and ulrastructural study of hemostasis after laser photocoagulation. Gastrointest Endosc 26: 131–133, 1980

12. Goff JS: Bipolar coagulation versus Neodymium-YAG laser photocoagulation for upper gastrointestinal bleeding lesions. Dig Dis Sci 31: 906–910, 1986

13. Goudie BM, Mitchell KG, Birnie GG, Mackey C: Controlled trial of endoscopic bipolar electrocoagulation in the treatment of bleeding peptic ulcers. Gut 25: A1185, 1984

14. Griffiths WJ, Neumann DA, Welsh JD: The visible vessel as an indicator of uncontrolled or recurrent gastrointestinal hemorrhage. N Engl J Med 300: 411–413, 1979

15. Hirao M, Kobayaski T, Masuda K, et al: Endoscopic local injection of hypertonic saline-epinephrine solution to arrest hemorrhage from the upper gastrointestinal tract. Gastrointest Endosc 31: 313–317, 1985

16. Ihre T, Johansson C, Seligson U, et al: Endoscopic Y.A.G. laser treatment in massive upper gastrointestinal bleeding. Scand. J Gastroenterol 16: 633–640, 1981

17. Johnston J, Stones J, Long B: Heater probe is superior to YAG laser in clinical endoscopic treatment of major bleeding from peptic ulcers. Gastrointest Endosc 30: 154–156, 1984

18. Kernohan RM, Anderson JR, McKelvey STD, Kennedy TL: A controlled trial of bipolar electrocoagulation in patients with upper gastrointestinal bleeding. Br J Surg 71: 889–891, 1984

19. Kiefhaber P: Endoscopic applications of Nd:YAG laser radiation in the gastrointestinal tract. In: Joffe SN (ed.): Neodymium-YAG Laser Medicine and Surgery. New York, Elsevier, 1983 (pp 6–14)

20. Kiefhaber P, Nath G, Moritz K: Endoscopic control of irradiation with a high power neodymium YAG laser. Prog Surg 15: 140–145, 1977

21. Krejs, GJ, Little KH, Westergaard H, et al: Laser photocoagulation for the treatment of acute peptic ulcer bleeding: A randomized controlled clinical trial. Gastroenterology 88: 1457, 1985

22. Laine L: A controlled trial of multipolar electrocoagulation in the treatment of the upper gastrointestinal hemorrhage. New England J Med 316: 1613–1617, 1987

23. McLeod I, Mills PR, MacKenzie JF, et al: Neodymium YAG-laser photocoagulation for major hemorrhage from peptic ulcers and single vessels. Br Med J 286: 345–348, 1983

24. Rutgeerts P, Broeckaert L, Coremans G, Janssens J, Van Isveldt J, Vantrappen G: Randomized comparison of three hemostasis modalities for severely bleeding peptic ulcers: Epinephrin 1‰ injection alone (1), epinephrin + polidocanol 1% injection (2), epinephrin injection followed by YAG laser (3). Gastrointest Endosc 33: 182, 1987

25. Rutgeerts P, Geboes K, Vantrappen G: Tissue damage produced by haemostatic injections. Gastrointest Endosc 32: 179,1986

26. Rutgeerts P, Vantrappen G, Broeckaert L: A new and effective technique of YAG laser photocoagulation for severe upper gastrointestinal bleeding. Endoscopy 16: 115–117, 1984

27. Rutgeerts P, Vantrappen G, Broeckaert L, Janssens J, Coremans G, Geboes K, Schurmans P: Controlled trial of YAG laser treatment of upper digestive hemorrhage. Gastroenterology 83: 410–416, 1982

28. Rutgeerts P, Vantrappen G, Geboes K: Safety and efficacy of Neodymium-Yag laser photocoagulation – an experimental study in dogs. Gut 22: 38–44, 1981

29. Rutgeerts P, Vantrappen G, Geboes K, Broekkaert L: Neodymium-Yag laser photocoagulation for hemostasis of gastrointestinal non-variceal hemorrhage. Z Gastroenterol 21: 263–267, 1983

30. Rutgeerts P, Vantrappen G, Van Hootegem Ph, Broeckaert L, Janssens J, Coremans G, Geboes K: Neodymium-YAG laser photocoagulation versus multipolar electrocoagulation for the treatment of severely bleeding peptic ulcers: A randomized comparison. Gastrointest Endosc. 33, 199–202, 1987

31. Sander R, Pösl H, Spuhler A, Hitzler H: Der Neodymium-Yag-Laser: Ein effectives Instrument für die Stillung lebensbedrohlicher Gastrointestinalblutungen. Leber Magen Darm 11: 31–36, 1981

32. Schiller KFR, Truelove SG, Williams DG: Haematemesis and malaena, with special reference to factors influencing outcome. Br Med J 2: 7–14, 1970

33. Shönekäs: Personal communication

34. Silverstein FE, Gilbert DA, Tedesco FJ, et al: The national ASGE survey on upper gastrointestinal bleeding. Parts 1–3. Gastrointest Endosc 27: 73–102, 1982

35. Soehendra N: Sclerotherapy of upper gastrointestinal haemorrhage. Z Gastroenterol 21: 259–262, 1983

36. Storey DW, Bown SG, Swain CP: Endoscopic prediction of recurrent bleeding of peptic ulcers N Engl J Med 305: 915–916, 1981

37. Swain CP, Bown SG, Salmon PR, et al: Controlled trial of neodymium YAG laser photocoagulation in bleeding peptic ulcers. Lancet, 1986; 1: 1113–1117

38. Swain CP, Storey DW, Bown SG, Heath J, Mills TN, Salmon PR, Nortfield TC, Kirkham JS, O'Sullivan JP: Nature of the bleeding vessel in recurrently bleeding gastric ulcers. Gastroenterology 90: 595–608, 1986

39. Wara P: Endoscopic prediction of major rebleeding – a prospective study of stigmata of hemorrhage in bleeding ulcers. Gastroenterology 88: 1209–1214, 1985

Palliative Therapy of Malignant Tumors

J. F. Riemann, B. Kohler, and C. Ell

In recent years, palliative treatment of malignant stenoses of the upper gastrointestinal tract has been considerably enriched by laser therapy (1–4, 7, 12, 14, 15, 18–20). Before this, such effective procedures as endoscopic bougienage and the implantation of an esophageal tube were available; in addition, apart from palliative surgical resection and surgical tube placement, chemotherapy, radiotherapy, and percutaneous endoscopic gastrostomy, were also used (Table 1). The disadvantages of most of these procedures are the relatively high rates of associated complications and mortality, their frequently complicated nature, the considerable time requirement, and poor acceptance by the patient in the individual case. Many of these disadvantages have now been eliminated by laser therapy.

Laser System

We make use of a neodymium:yttrium-aluminum-garnet (Nd:YAG) laser (Medilas II, MBB/Ottobrunn) (Fig. 1). At a wavelength of 1064 nm, it delivers a power output of up to 110 W. As a transmission system, this laser is provided with a monofibre with coaxial carbon dioxide flow, and an apical metal jet. The fiber has a diameter of 2.6 mm. As the carrier endoscope, we use instruments manufactured by the firm of Olympus (GIF XQ 10, prototype GF Q 10 with a 3.5 mm channel and prototype GIF Q 10, which is made of white material, for use in the upper gastrointestinal tract). The routine laser gastroscope should generally be provided with a white ceramic or Teflon cap to prevent burning of the tip of the endoscope (Fig. 2) (15).

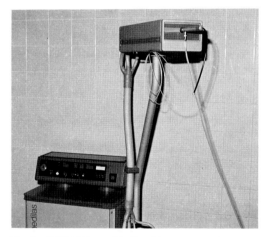

Fig. 1 Nd:YAG laser (Medilas 2).

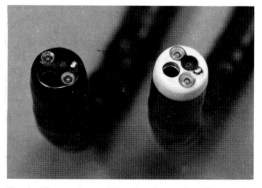

Fig. 2 Comparison of the tip of a routine fiber endoscope (black) and the white ceramic tip.

Table 1 Procedures for the Palliative Treatment of Malignant Tumors of the Upper Gastrointestinal Tract

Surgical resection, surgical tube placement
Radiotherapy
Chemotherapy
Endoscopic bougienage
Endoscopic tube placement
Percutaneous endoscopic gastrostomy
Endoscopic laser treatment

Preparation

All our patients are premedicated before the procedure. This premedication is dictated by experience, since, occasionally, the development of heat can give rise to painful sensations. In common with many other procedures, the premedication improves patient acceptance of the technique. Essentially, it consists of 50 to 100 mg pethidin or 2.5 to 10 mg midazolam given with the aim of reducing the motility of the upper gastrointestinal tract.

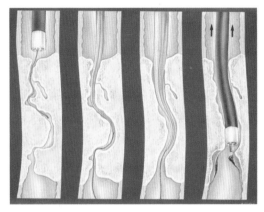

Fig. **3** Schematic drawing of the different steps of bougienage and laser vaporization.

Examination

As a rule, we work with a power output of 80 to 90 W. The total amount of energy applied varies individually per session between 1000 and 15,000 J.

The main aim of palliative tumor treatment is to recanalize the tumor-induced stenosis. This is particularly difficult to accomplish when virtually complete stenosis of the lumen is present. In such cases, it has proved expedient to use a combination of bougienage and laser therapy to accomplish the therapeutic objective more quickly (6, 7, 14). Under endoscopic visual control, a guide wire is carefully advanced through the tumor stenosis into the stomach (Fig. **3**). Bougienage is then performed using the Savary Gilliard bougie or the Eder Puestow bougie to a degree that permits the subsequent passage of the endoscope. As a rule, the diameter of the recanalized lumen is between 1.2 and 1.4 cm. At the same session, or on the next day, the laser is used, in a circular fashion, working from the caudad to the cranial direction, with a distance to the object of about 0.5 to 1.0 cm, to vaporize the tumorous tissue (Figs. **4–6**). If the entrance of the tumor stenosis is very narrow, or if it is of a cufflike nature, it is recommended that this entrance obstacle first be eliminated. Lately, a laser-resistant guide probe has been developed, along which va-

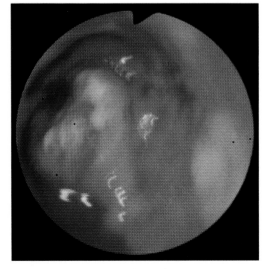

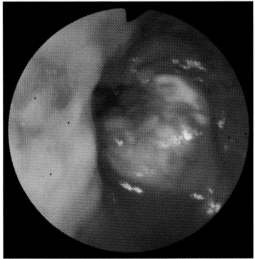

Fig. **4** Esophageal tumor obstruction.

porization of the tumor without prior bougienage is possible (5).

The success of opening tumor stenoses can
be demonstrated additionally, of course, by
radiology (Fig. **7a, b**); however, in some cases
this is not as impressive as by endoscopy.

In many cases, a step by step dilation of
the stenosis in a number of individual sessions
is necessary (14, 18, 19). Necrotic tissue can be

removed either with the instrument itself or
with the aid of additional instruments, such as
a diathermy loop or basket.

In all cases, immediate postoperative
radiologic monitoring (diatrizoate meglumine
swallow) is required in order to be able to
recognize and treat any complications, in particular, perforation, in good time. Even perforations after laser vaporization are initially

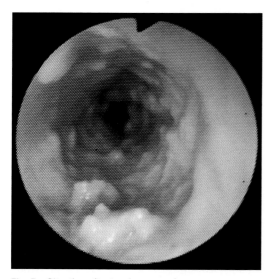
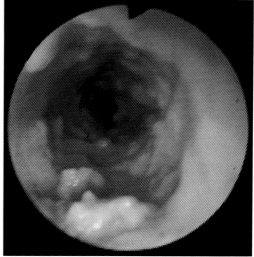

Fig. **5**   Situation after two laser sessions.

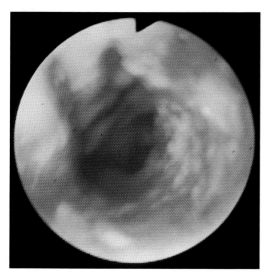
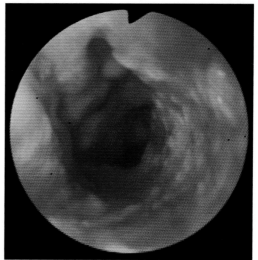

Fig. **6**   Tumor stenosis completely recanalized.

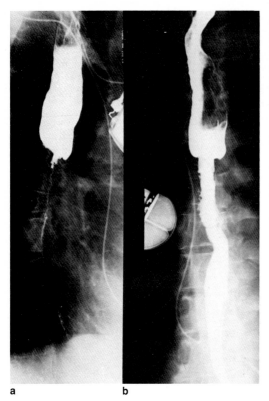

a   b

Fig. **7** Esophageal carcinoma **a** before and **b** after laser therapy.

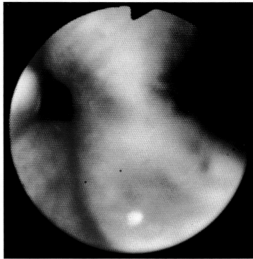

Fig. **8** Leakage to the mediastinum after laser therapy.

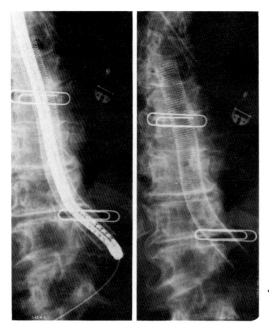

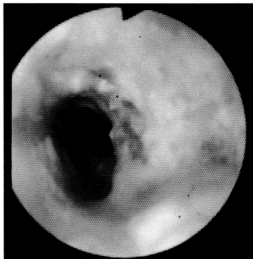

Fig. **9** Successful closure with Ethibloc.

◀Fig. **10** Endoscopically implanted endoprosthesis after an unsuccessful trial to close a fistula by blocking agents.

treatable by conservative means, as in similar cases of iatrogenic perforation due to other endoscopic maneuvers. In the case of small fistulas, an attempt can be made, using rapidly hardening amino acid solutions (for example, Ethibloc) or fibrin adhesive (Figs, **8, 9**), to seal off the leak (13, 16). If this does not succeed, a tube must be placed (Fig. **10**).

Results

In the period between April 1, 1985, and March 31, 1987, we treated a total of 47 patients with inoperable malignant stenoses of the upper gastrointestinal tract. These included 27 carcinomas of the esophagus and 16 carcinomas of the cardia, three recurrent stenoses after carcinomas of the larynx, and a single case of hypernephroma that had metastasized to the esophagus. Thirty-four patients were male and 13 were female. Further details are given in Table **2**. On the average, the intervals between treatment sessions were approximately 5 to 8 weeks, with a range between 14 days and 4 months. The mean observation time of the patients with carcinoma of the esophagus was 5.3 months (1 to 16 months), that of cases of gastric carcinoma was 8.7 months (2 to 21 months).

In all patients, the passage was reestablished after the first session to such a degree that at least adequate enteral liquid alimentation was possible. The actual objective of the treatment, that is, the reestablishment of normal eating habits involving the intake of solid food, proved to be achievable in 78.7% of the patients (Table **3**). On the average, patients with esophageal stenoses required 3.4 sessions and patients with gastric carcinoma, 2.6 sessions.

Complications

The rate of complications in our series was extremely small. We observed a single case of septic complication in a patient in whom a hypernephroma had metastasized to the esophagus (9). No case of direct perforation after laser therapy was observed; the sole perforation that was seen occurred subsequent to irridation (Table **4**).

Table **2** Patient Data (from Medical Department C, Municipal Hospital, Ludwigshafen)

Location (of Tumor, Stenosis)	Patients	Age (Years; Range)
Esophagus		
Upper third	8	
Middle third	14	55.3 (43–81)
Lower third	9	
Total	31	
Stomach		
Cardia	14	
Body	2	72.6 (60–79)
Total	16	
Total	47	

Table **4** Complications (from the Medical Department C, Municipal Hospital Ludwigshafen)

Localization	Complication	Deaths
Esophagus	2*/31 (6.4%)	1**/31 (3.2%)
Stomach	0/16	–
Total	2/47 (4.2%)	1/47 (2.1%)

  * 1 perforation, 1 sepsis
 ** sepsis

Table **3** Observation Period Success Rate* (from the Medical Department C, Municipal Hospital, Ludwigshafen)

Localisation	Treatment Successful	Observation Period (Mo; Range)	No. of Therapies
Esophagus	27/31 (87.1%)	5.3 (1–14)	3.4 (1–16)
Stomach	10/16 (62.5%)	8.7 (2–21)	2.6 (1– 8)
Total	37/47 (78.7%)		

 * Solid food can be taken

Table 5   Results of Palliative Laser Therapy in the Upper Gastrointestinal Tract (from the Department of Internal Medicine, University of Erlangen; May 1. 1984, to March 31, 1987)

Location	Patients (no.)	Age (Y)	Number of Sessions (no.)	Success Rate*	Complications	Death
Esophagus						
Upper third	15			53/66	3/66	1/66
Middle third	24			(80.3%)	(4.5%)	(1.5%)
Lower third	27					
Stomach						
Cardia	53			52/66	1/66	
Body	13			(78.7%)	(1.5%)	
Total	132	66.9	2.4	105/132	4/132	1/132
Range		25–95	1–9	79.5%	3.03%	0.75%

* Oral nutrition (solid food) possible

Results of the Erlangen group are summarized in Table 5 and are in good agreement with the presented data.

Discussion

Today, there is no disputing concerning the fact that laser therapy is a highly effective and efficient therapeutic procedure for the rapid elimination of obstructing malignant processes in the upper digestive tract (2, 7, 8, 15, 17). In large series, the technique has been shown to be associated with relatively few complications compared with the other palliative measures (11). This experience is also very impressively confirmed in a survey involving a large number of centers (6). Used in combination with bougienage, a free passage can quickly be reestablished, often under outpatient conditions. Laser therapy is simple in application, requires little time, and is readily tolerated by the patient. In our experience, patients who have undergone such treatment and who are able to compare it with other therapeutic procedures, favor this technique over the other measures. The main reason for this is the fact that one of the vital functions, oral alimentation, becomes possible in many cases immediately after laser treatment. In particular, the foreign body sensation and the fetid smell associated with the tube prosthesis are obviated.

The success of laser treatment depends quite decisively on the length of the stenosis, the depth of tumor infiltration, and a possible associated infiltration of neural structures, which may be responsible for additional disturbances of motility. Thus, in the individual case, it may have to be established why, in the presence of a free passage, normal alimentation is still not possible.

Difficulties are always encountered when a very sharp angulation is present in the region of the cardia. It is possible that the danger of perforation can be drastically reduced with the aid of the laserresistant guide probe. Otherwise, it must be carefully considered whether the placement of a short tube prosthesis might not be preferable to laser treatment. Recently, we have begun to employ a gastroscope made of white material (prototype GIF Q 10, white). With the aid of this instrument, the cardia can be treated close to the instrument, even in inversion; the shaft is protected from destruction by the (reduced) absorption of the laser ligth by the white material.

We have obtained extremely good results with laser therapy, in particular in the case of tumors located high up in the esophagus. The laser is often the sole possible form of treatment in such cases, since a prosthesis is difficult to place and is also associated with many disadvantages (10). This has been confirmed most impressively in a patient who, after neck dissection for a carcinoma of the larynx, developed a malignant recurrent stenosis in the upper esophagus. Because of a rigorous combination of bougienage and laser treatment, a free passage that permitted regular alimentation has now been maintained for the past 12 months, with only local tumor growth. The lumen in this patient is dilated at regular intervals.

A negative aspect of laser therapy, apart from the question of cost, is, in particular, the need for frequent applications of the laser. Whenever this can be done on an outpatient basis, the economic factor may be neglected. As a rule, the dysphagia-free interval varies between 4 and 8 weeks. The result is that patients have to consult their physician relatively frequently and have to undergo repeated treatment. Experience has, however, shown that the widespread use of laser treatment, also in small hospitals, has resulted in the fact that, since the operator of the laser equipment often lacks sufficient experience, the possibilities of this form of treatment are not being utilized to the full and the dysphagia-free interval is thereby unnessesarily shortened.

Whether additional intracavitary irradiation might appreciably lengthen the dysphagia-free interval remains a matter for further study.

Conclusions

In recent years, palliative laser treatment of malignant strictures and stenoses of the upper gastrointestinal tract has won a place over all the other therapeutic procedures available. It cannot, however, be used when esophago-tracheal fistulas are present, or when, in the case of carcinoma of the cardia, an unfavorable angulation is encountered. It can used after placement of a prosthetic tube, when the tube has become obstructed by tumor overgrowth in combination with a low power contact tip of sopphire or metal. A warning must, however, be given against the uncritical use of the laser. The decision to use laser therapy must be preceded by a careful diagnostic evaluation of the situation in order to avoid robbing the patient of the chance of a possibly curative procedure.

References

1. Bass M: Lasers for use in medicine. Endoscopy 18: 2, 1986

2. Buset M, Dunham F, Baize M, Toeuf J de, Cremer M: Nd-YAG-laser, a new palliative alternative in the management of esophageal cancer. Endoscopy 15: 353, 1983
3. Dwyer RM: The technique of gastrointestinal laser endoscopy. In: Goldman, L (ed): The Biomedical Laser. Springer, New York 1981
4. Dwyer, RM: The history of gastrointestinal endoscopic laser hemostasis and management. Endoscopy 18: 10, 1986
5. Ell C, Hochberger J, Lux G, Riemann JF: Laser-resistant guide probe for laser treatment of endoscopically impassable tumour stenoses. Endoscopy 18: 27, 1986
6. Ell C, Riemann JF, Lux G, Demling L: Palliative laser treatment of malignant stenoses in the upper gastrointestinal tract. Endoscopy 18: 21, 1986
7. Fleischer D: The laser in gastroenterology with emphasis on upper gastrointestinal malignancies. Gastrointest Endosc 33: 119, 1987
8. Fleischer D, Sivak Jr MV: Endoscopic Nd: YAG laser therapy as palliation for esophagogastric cancer. Gastroenterology 89: 827, 1985
9. Kohler B, Ginsbach C, Riemann JF: Bakteriämien nach endoskopischer Lasertherapie. Fortschr Med 4: 61, 1987
10. Lux G, Riemann JF, Groitl H: Endoskopische Palliativtherapie beim Ösophaguskarzinom. Fortschr Med 102: 285, 1984
11. Mathus-Vliegen EMH: Complications and pitfalls of laser therapy. Endoscopy 18: 69, 1986
12. Riemann JF: Lasertherapie im Gastrointestinaltrakt. Internist Prax 26: 645, 1986
13. Riemann JF, Ell C: Endoskopischer Verschluß einer tumorbedingten ösophago-mediastinalen Fistel mit einer schnell härtenden Aminosäurelösung. Dtsch Med. Wochenschr. 110: 396, 1985
14. Riemann JF, Ell C, Lux G, Demling L: Combined therapy of malignant stenoses of the upper gastrointestinal tract by means of laser beam and bougienage. Endoscopy 2: 43, 1985
15. Riemann JF, Kohler B: Behandlung mit Laserstrahlen im Verdauungstrakt. Fortschr Med 27–28: 525, 1986
16. Riemann JF, Nowack G: Tumorfistelokklusion im Rektum mit Ethibloc. Dtsch Med Wochenschr. 110: 1592, 1985
17. Riemann JF, Weber J, Kohler B: Ablation of a gastric neurogenic tumor with endoscopic laser therapy. Gastrointest. Endosc 33: 266, 1987
18. Sander R, Poesl H, Spuhler A: Therapie gastrointestinaler Tumoren mit Laser. Internist (Berlin) 26: 22, 1985
19. Sander R, Poesl H: Endoskopische Lasertherapie. Leber Magen Darm 6: 234, 1985
20. Unsöld E: Möglichkeiten und Grenzen des Lasers. Verhandlungsbericht Internistenkongreß 1986

Benign Stenoses

R. Sander

The neodymium:aluminum-garnet (Nd:YAG) laser has been used for treating non-neoplastic stenoses since 1983 (7). Although we are still optimistic regarding laser application in lower gastrointestinal tract indications, limited definitive long-term results of laser treatment in the upper gastrointestinal tract have given rise to viewing this method today in a more realistic light. Nevertheless, laser coagulation has to be taken into consideration when all competitive methods already known are too risky or do not reveal satisfactory results in a patient requiring treatment for a stricture in the upper gastrointestinal tract.

Between July 1983 and April 1987, 21 patients with non-neoplastic stenoses of the upper gastrointestinal tract were treated with the laser (Table **1**). Indications for this therapy were considered to be symptomatic strictures that could not be passed with the shaft of a routine endoscope of 13 mm in diameter caused by thickening of the wall of the organ. The cause of the strictures included reflux, peptic ulcer disease, caustic burn, postoperative scarring of an anastomosis and sclerotherapy.

Method

The Nd:YAG laser (type Medilas 2, MBB, Ottobrunn, FRG) with continuous wave (cw) mode, 1064 nm (and 1318 nm), and maximum power output 110 W (40 W) was used.

Transmission system was a noncontact quartz monofiber 0.6 mm in diameter with a Teflon cover, coaxial carbon dioxide flow, apical metal jet. Diameter of the whole system was 2.0 to 2.8 mm, with transmission of 90 to 100 W (30 to 35 W). Shooting distance from tip to target tissue was 5 mm. The effect of the laser beam was observed continuously during the treatment with shots of no fixed time limitation.

Olympus (GIF Q 10 and ACM FX 8) endoscopes were used.

Technique

Vaporization or coagulation of the scar ring or stenosis was carried out to a depth of 1 to 2 mm in the wall of the organ. The step by step photocoagulation begins at the margin of the stricture close to the tip of the endoscope. During a single session, two points or longitu-

Table **1**   Laser Treatment of Endoscopically not Passable Stenoses in the Upper Gastrointestinal Tract*

Localization	Cause	Patients	Patients with Repeated Laser Treatments
Esophagus	Reflux	6	5
	Sclerotherapy	3	2
	Caustic burn	2	2
Stomach	Surgery (anastomosis)	6	2
	Peptic ulcer disease, caustic burn	1	1
Duodenum	Peptic ulcer disease	2	1
		21	13

* From July 1983 to April 1987

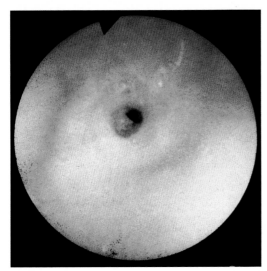

Fig. **1**   Nearly complete stenosis of the distal part of the esophagus, caused by reflux esophagitis.

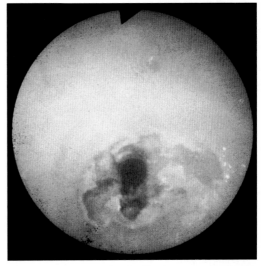

Fig. **2**   Immediately after the first laser treatment, with cuts in contralateral positions. The peripheral lesions are mucosa defects after contact with the tip of the endoscope.

dinal strips up to a maximum of 2 to 3 cm in length on opposite positions of the stenosis are vaporized. During the first session, no additional bougienage should be done because of the risk of uncontrolled rupture of the organic wall.

An endoscopic follow-up was done 2 to 3 days later. If necessary, a new treatment session was carried out, in some cases with additional bougienage with the endoscope. Power was 90 to 100 W (30 to 35 W).

The total amount of energy applied depended on the structure and the extent of the stricture, e. g., Schatzki ring 200 J, long peptic stenosis up to 10,000 J per session. The goal of the treatment was palliative, if possible, curative, reopening of the narrowing to allow easy passage with the 13 mm endoscope. This passage is usually sufficient to eliminate dysphagia. In all cases repeated treatments and follow-ups are necessary.

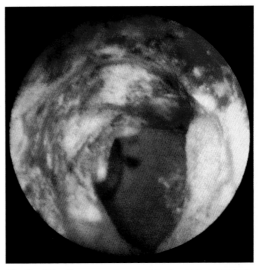

Fig. **3**   After three sessions within 1 week, a passage for the 13 mm endoscope is possible. Patient is a 61-year-old man. Stenosis 25 to 31 cm from the teeth row, lumen before treatment was 2 to 3 mm.

Results

All stenoses were primarily treated sucessfully, reopened for a passage with the 13 mm endoscope, which proved to be nesessary for the elimination of dysphagia.

Stenoses due to *reflux* in six (four women, two men) patients 61 to 80 years of age (mean age 74.2 years) were treated in 82 sessions.

One short stenosis (10 mm) only needed one treatment. The other five stenoses were 3 to 9 cm of length (mean, 5.6 cm). Each of those patients needed 16.2 sessions in a treatment period of up to 21 months to keep the passage passable for the 13 mm endoscope (Figs. **1–3**).

One of the six patients died from a severe underlying heart disease, one underwent surgical resection, two are still in treatment, and two patients are cured. Follow-up time was 9 to 45 months (mean, 29.7).

Stenoses due to *sclerotherapy* in three (two women, one man) patients, 40 to 44 years of age, were treated in 11 sessions. Length of the strictures was 3 to 6 cm (mean, 4.8). One patient needed to be treated only once to achieve a good result (follow-up, 17 months). One woman is still undergoing treatment (once every 2 months) and one female patient died from variceal bleeding between two laser sessions. In this single case only of 21 patients, most of them inoperable, a complication was observed that is due to the whole therapeutic concept of treating esophageal varices, including laser coagulation. The female patient with almost complete stenosis of the distal third of the esophagus after sclerotherapy was in a very poor clinical condition, with known decompensated alcoholic cirrhosis of the liver and hepatic precoma. Two days after successful treatment of the stenosis with the laser, a spurting hemorrhage from the esophagocardial junction occured. Attempts to accomplish hemostasis with the laser resulted in a perforation that led to the death of the patient within a matter of days.

Stenoses from *caustic burns* were treated in three patients (two of them female) 13, 19, and 66 years of age. In two of them we achieved a definitive reopening of the esophagus/pyloric region after five to six treatments within 6 weeks. Length of the stenoses was 3 to 4 cm. One 13-year-old female patient was treated several times, successfully opening up a stenosis of initially 3 cm, later 6 cm in length. Finally, we decided to perform surgery (colon interposition) to achieve a definite cure (Figs. **4, 5**).

Peptic ulcer disease had caused strictures in two men and a woman, 32, 74 and 78 years old. We reopened the scarring with laser coagulation. The length of the stenoses was 2 cm on average. In one case definitive reopening was possible within 1 session. In the other two cases after 1 successful reopening within two to five sessions later, an elective surgery was performed to cure the chronic peptic ulcer disease.

Postoperative scarring of an anastomosis after partial or complete stomach resection

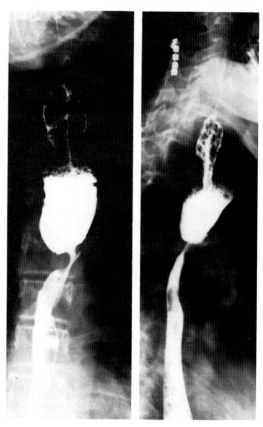

Fig. 4 13-Year-old female patient with a 2 cm long stricture in the proximal part of the esophagus after drinking lye at the age of 2 years. Radiograph shows the extent and degree of the stricture.

was treated in six patients (five men, one woman), 49 to 80 years of age (mean, 69.2) with strictures 0.5 to 3 cm in length (mean, 1.9 cm). Three patients were cured after a single session; in one patient a recurrent carcinoma was revealed in biopsies 6 months later after a first recanalization. One patient needed five sessions for a definitive good result. Only in one patient a surgical intervention followed a period of 12 laser treatments done within 4 months. The follow-up of the patients with only laser treatment continued for 5 to 35 months (mean, 17.3). Of three patients in whom we initially suspected a non-neoplastic stenosis of the esophagus, one subsequently proved to have recurrent and two had primary carcinoma. These patients were excluded from this study.

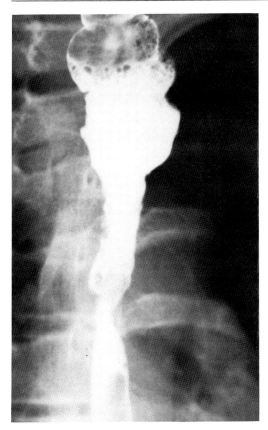

Fig. **5** Same patient as Figure **4**. After the first treatment, a good primary result was achieved.

Discussion

Severe dysphagia in patients with a narrow non-neoplastic stenosis of the upper gastrointestinal tract demands therapy sufficient to prevent undernutrition and infection due to lung aspiration. In common with other surgical interventions involving general anesthesia, surgical treatment of such a stricture entails a certain risk, in particular for patients with restricted operability. Disadvantages of the well-known conservative methods, i. e., bougienage, are the only short-term effects with frequent recurrences, and the possibility of complications, in particular ruptures and perforations (8, 9). With all bougies, benign strictures need to be retreated at short intervals for the rest of the patients' lives (12, 5). Other methods did not reveal better efficacy in

our experience (3, 4). Being on the lookout for an effective endoscopic operative method with safe and easy handling, the Nd:YAG laser proved to be an excellent and practicable means of opening up cicatrizing and inflammatory endoscopically accessible strictures of the gastrointestinal tract (6).

All non-neoplastic stenoses of the gastrointestinal tract with a thickening of the wall are suitable for laser treatment. Basically, nearly all of them can be primarily treated with success. The effectiveness of the laser treatment depends on the localization, extent, and cause of the stricture. Stenoses of the lower gastrointestinal tract are easier to handle. In the upper gastrointestinal tract, gastric acid often plays a role in the development of a renarrowing of a laser-treated lesion, with its defects of the mucosa and submucosa. The longer a stenosis, the more it tends to recur. In the case of a short stenosis, especially a Schatzki ring or a web, a single session usually suffices to achieve a cure.

Similar good results can be successfully accomplished in short postoperative scarred anastomic strictures, i. e., after partial or complete resection of the stomach, if they are less than 2 to 3 cm in length.

Long strictures that are primarily supposedly benign, are always suspicious of a carcinoma, even when repeated forceps biopsies fail to reveal any malignancy. This is of particular importance when, during the course of the treatment, a stenosis increases in length, especially in the distal part of the esophagus in a peptic stenosis or in the region of an anastomosis after resection of a carcinoma. The increase in the length of the stricture, together with a shortening of the intervals between treatment sessions, are indicative of malignancy.

In narrowing caused by inflammatory processes, the dynamics of the underlying disease determine the tendency of the stenosis to recur.

It is evident that in patients with long peptic stenoses or strictures caused by caustic burns good results are difficult to obtain. Furthermore, they are considered to be precancerous lesions. Laser coagulation and complementary bougienage with the fiber endoscope should be restricted to inoperable patients and must be repeated at increasingly lengthy intervals, to stabilize the initial results of treatment under the usual adjuvant therapy using suitable drugs (H_2-blocking agents, antacids, etc.).

In cases of frequent recurrences or long stenoses of more than 3 cm in length, operable patients should, whenever possible, be submitted to surgery, even when repeated biopsies do not reveal malignancy. Because perforation and bleeding remain a certain hazard of every endoscopic operative procedure, the use of the Nd:YAG laser should be restricted to patients with symptoms (dysphagia) who are not suspected of having an operable cancer. Whenever there is an indication for an endoscopic operative treatment of a symptomatic non-neoplastic stenosis, the Nd:YAG laser should be considered as the method of choice. In many cases unnecessary surgery is obviated, the quality of the patient's life is improved.

References

1. Burkhart K, Sullican B: Course and treatment of benign esophageal strictures. Am J Gastroenterol 58: 531, 1972

2. Davis WM, Madden J, Peacock E: A new approach to the control of esophageal stenosis. Am Surg 176: 469, 1972

3. Groitl H: Endoscopic treatment of scar stenosis in the upper GI tract. Endoscopy 16: 165, 1984

4. Lindor K, Ott B, Hughes R: Ballon dilatation of upper digestive tract strictures. Gastroenterology 89: 545, 1985

5. Price J, Stancin C, Bennett R: A safer method of dilating esophageal strictures. Lancet 1: 1141, 1974

6. Sander R, Poesl H: Treatment of non-neoplastic stenoses with the ND-YAG laser – indications and limitations. Endoscopy 18 (Suppl 1): 53, 1986

7. Sander H, Poesl H, Spuhler A: Management of non-neoplastic stenoses of the GI tract – a further indication for Nd YAG laser application. Endoscopy 16: 149, 1984

8. Wesdorp K, Bertelsman J, Den Hartog Jager F, Huibregtse K, Tytgat G: Results of conservative treatment of benign esophageal stricture. A follow-up study in 100 patients. Gastroenterology 8: 487, 1982

9. Williamson R: The management of peptic esophageal strictures. Br J Surg 62: 445, 1975

Early Gastric Cancer

T. Takemoto, Y. Okazaki, H. Fujimura, T. Otani, I. Tanabe, and Y. Fukumoto

Laser endoscopy was developed with the hemostatic therapy of upper gastrointestinal bleeding in the field of gastroenterology in mind. Since the first case of laser therapy for early gastric cancer was reported in 1978 (2), laser endoscopy has been applied in Japan more frequently for the treatment of cancer than for hemostasis (1). Therefore we report the present usefulness and problems in laser therapy for early gastric cancer in Japan.

Status of Laser Therapy in Gastric Cancer in Japan

Radical operation is the treatment of first choice for gastric cancer. However, cancer patients are not always suitable for surgical treatment because of accompanying severe respiratory and cardiac diseases, and advanced age. Laser therapy in gastric cancer is limited to such cases.

In the analysis of the questionaire concerning laser therapy performed by the Laser Comittee of Japanese Gastroenterological Endoscopic Society, 1573 cases with gastrointestinal tract cancer were treated by laser endoscopy aimed at curative or palliative treatment until November 1985, as shown in Table 1. In Japan, curativ therapy accounted for 1091 cases, and the ratio of gastric cancer was 91%.

Among the patients with gastric cancer receiving laser therapy, 867 of 978 cases (89%) were early gastric cancer. Of this group, 364 cases (42%) could be followed up by endoscopy with biopsy continuously and the therapy was histologically confirmed as curative for more than a 1-year period after laser irradiation. On the other hand, recurrence was observed in 95 of 867 cases (11%). The follow-up in the remaining 408 cases was too short to evaluate the therapeutic effect, although they included no recurrence.

Table 1 Laser Endoscopic Treatment for Gastrointestinal Cancer in Japan

Laser Endoscopic Treatment	Object	Cases
Curative treatment	Esophageal cancer	54
	Gastric cancer	978
	Colon cancer	52
	Duodenal cancer	7
Subtotal		1091
Symptomatic treatment	Bleeding	102
	Stenosis	327
	Other	53
Subtotal		482
Total		1573

Our Experience with Laser Therapy for Early Gastric Cancer

Endoscopic laser therapy for early gastric cancer was started in December 1980 in our institution.

The MBB neodymium:yttrium-aluminum-garnet (Nd:YAG) laser and Aloka LMY 1001 YAG laser were used as laser coagulators. Machida FGS-L and Olympus Q, Q10 were used as endoscopes, and quartz fiber for transmission of laser. The conditions of laser irradiation were 40 to 60 W of power, 0.5 to 1.0 s irradiation time, and 1.5 to 2.0 cm distance from the tip of the quartz fiber to the tissue.

The diagnosis of early gastric cancer was made by both endoscopy with biopsy and radiography. The subjects for laser therapy were patients who were diagnosed as having early gastric cancer, but were not feasible for surgical treatment due to secondary illnesses or advance age.

The therapeutic effect of this treatment for early gastric cancer in our institution is shown in Table **2**. The total number of patients irradiated by laser were 48 cases with 54 lesions, from December 1980 to August 1986. One patient died of exacerbation of other accompanying diseases in the days following laser therapy, and another patient is still in laser treatment. So our follow-up includes 52 lesions in 46 cases.

Six lesions in six cases were operated on within 1 year after laser therapy because their other illnesses improved to a point acceptable for surgical treatment. In only one case of surgical therapy were cancer cells found in the wall of the stomach during the histologic examination.

In a period of 1 year following endoscopic bite biopsy after laser irradiation, 42 lesions in 40 cases were negative for cancer cells; in four cases cancer cells remained. Repeated laser therapy was initiated in these four cases of recurrence. After reirradiation, no recurrence of cancer was detected in three cases by bite biopsy during the term of observation, but one patient died of aggravation of accompanying diseases soon after reirradiation.

Table **3** shows the diagnosis of the patients with no recurrence of gastric cancer in the period following first irradiation. In 42 lesions of 36 cases, six patients with nine lesions died of other accompanying diseases, but in all surviving patients no recurrence was observed in endoscopic bite biopsy.

The incidence of recurrence in this study was evaluated in relationship to size, macroscopic type, histologic type, and depth of invasion of the tumor. Results showed that the therapeutic effect could be related to the size of the lesion: laser irradiation was more effective in lesions less than 2 cm in diameter (Table **4**).

Early gastric cancer can be classified into three types; elevated, flat, and depressed. As shown in Table **5**, in the elevated type, that is, I or IIa, all cases were free of the cancer after laser therapy. On the other hand, in the depressed type, that is, IIc or IIc+III, recurrence was noted in 14% of the cases during the follow-up period. It appeared that such results might depend on the unclear identification of invasion in the depressed type.

In the study of the histologic type of cancer, among lesions of the differentiated

Table **2** Results of Endoscopic Laser Therapy in Our Institution

	Operated Lesions	Follow-up Lesions
Cancer positive	1	4
Cancer negative	5	42
Total	6	46

Table **3** Follow-up Terms of Cancer-Negative Lesions after First Laser Irradiation

	Alive (Lesion)	Died of Other Disease (Lesion)
5 to 6 yr	1	
4 to 5 yr	7	1
3 to 4 yr	7	
2 to 3 yr	4	
1 to 2 yr	13	4
0 to 1 yr	1	4
Total	33	9

Table **4** Size of the Lesion and Results of Endoscopic Laser Therapy

Size	Cancer Negative (Continuously)	Cancer Positive (After First Irradiation)
3 to 4 cm		1
2 to 3 cm	5 (62%)	3
1 to 2 cm	24 (96%)	1
0 to 1 cm	18 (100%)	
Total	46 (90%)	5

Table **5** Macrosopic Type and Results of Laser Therapy

Macroscopic Type	Cancer Negative (Continuously)	Cancer Positive (After First Irradiation)
Elevated	15 (100%)	0
Depressed	32 (86%)	5 (14%)
Total	47 (90%)	5 (10%)

Table **6** Depth of Invasion and Results of Laser Therapy

Depth of Invasion	Cancer Negative (Continuously)	Cancer Positive (After First Irradiation)
m	31 (100%)	0
sm	16 (76%)	5 (24%)
Total	47 (90%)	5 (10%)

type, 96% of cases were negative after first laser irradiation. In the undifferentiated type, recurrence was observed in 50% of cases. Thus, laser therapy was effective in the well-differentiated cancer. This result coincides with the fact that the elevated early gastric cancer almost always showed the well-differentiated histologic type.

Furthermore, the effect of laser was also studied in relation to depth of cancer invasions diagnosed by endoscopy and radiology. In the cases with type "m" early gastric cancer, in which cancer cells were located within the mucosal layer, no remaining cancer was detected after the first laser irradiation. In the type "sm" in which cancer invasion extended into the submucosa, recurrence was seen in 5 of 21 cases, as listed in Table **6**. It was concluded that for type "m" early cancer, laser therapy was very effective. This result also suggests that more sensitive diagnostic tools are needed for clarifying the depth of cancer invasion.

Problems in Laser Therapy for Early Gastric Cancer

As already mentioned, laser irradiation is very useful in the treatment of early gastric cancer, and this therapy is becoming rapidly popular in Japan. However, laser therapy as a curative treatment is still problematic.

Recurrent cases after laser irradiation accounted for 11% in the whole of Japan. We also had several cases of recurrence. The most important cause of recurrence is considered to be uncertain judgement of laser effect in the gastric wall. Especially in the depressed type of early gastric cancer, such as IIc or II+III, one tends to apply low laser energy in order to

avoid wall perforation. So, we will have to develop new clinical trials to ascertain laser effectiveness in the gastric wall.

The other problem is, this therapy is limited by several reasons to patients who are not admissable to surgery. For one reason, it is difficult to judge the metastasis to lymph nodes surrounding the stomach with the present diagnostic system. If cancer metastasis to lymph nodes could be detected in these cases, one could treat early gastric cancer more with laser without surgery.

New Approach in Laser Therapy to Early Gastric Cancer

We are not trying to use endoscopic ultrasonography (EUS) as a new approach for the problems discussed.

This apparatus has been developed in cooperation between Olympus Optical and Aloka Company in Japan. The tip of the endoscope is equipped with a 7.5 MHz transducer that can be rotated mechanically to produce an image covering a sector of 360°.

With this method, it has been reported that the five layers of the gastric wall can be clearly differentiated in the image (3). Thus, EUS may be applied to ascertain the effect of laser therapy. It shows the area of laser-irradiated gastric wall to be more echogenic than the nonirradiated area. EUS can also visualize the depth of invasion of gastric cancer as a sectional image of gastric wall. So it was actually possible in the patient with depressed-type early gastric cancer treated by laser, by using EUS, to obtain an image revealing a highly echogenic pattern in the submucosal layer that suggested the destruction of cancer nests.

Moreover, the lymph nodes surrounding the stomach can be detected in the echogram of EUS. Usually, these lymph nodes were visualized as low echogenic structures by EUS. Recently, an interesting trial has been attempted aiming at the image enhancement of the lymph nodes. It appears that normal lymph nodes become enhanced as highly echogenic structures in EUS after oral administration of sesame oil emulsion, but that metastatic cancerous lymph nodes are not enhanced.

As shown in Figure **1**, the lymph nodes without metastasis were visualized as highly echogenic structures after administration of the emulsion, but as shown in Figure **2**, the

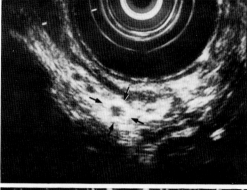

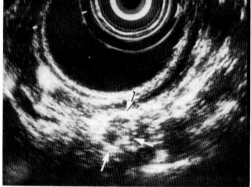

Fig. 1 The lymph node without metastasis was enhanced by sesame emulsion. The small (top) and larger (bottom) lymph nodes are indicated by arrows.

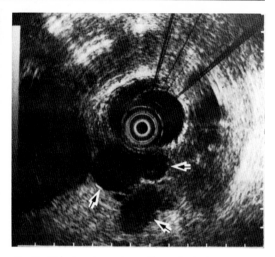

Fig. 2 The lymph nodes with metastasis were not enhanced by sesame emulsion. Arrows indicate the lymph nodes.

lymph nodes with cancer metastasis were not enhanced by the emulsion.

Summary

It appears that laser therapy in early gastric cancer is very effective. However, more accurate studies are needed. EUS examination should prove to be a tool for resolving this problem.

Moreover, the diagnosis of cancer metastasis to the lymph nodes might be one of the key points for the application of the endoscopic treatment. After overcoming these problems, endoscopic laser therapy to early gastric cancer could become more popular.

References

1. Mizushima K, Harada K, Okamura K, Matsuda T, Hayashi H, Namiki M, Kasai S, Mito M, Hara K, Atsumi K, Nishizaka K: Experimental investigation on the effects and safety of a laser coagulator and its application to clinical use. Gastroenterol Endosc 21: 938–947, 1979
2. Takemoto T: Laser therapy of early gastric cancer. Endoscopy 18 (Suppl): 33–36, 1986
3. Takemoto T, Aibe T, Fuji T, Okita K: Endoscopic ultrasonography. Clin Gastroenterol 15: 305–319, 1986

Biliary System

Papillotomy

R. Sander

Since the description of the first successful laser papillotomy on a patient with a stone in the common bile duct (5), laser treatment has revealed itself to be worth consideration in several further indications. When the well-known instruments and methods (2) are, for technical reasons, not sufficient to perform a sphincterotomy (the case in approximately 5% of patients without tumors or previous stomach resection [3]), laser light can be helpful for reopening of the orifice. We have tested it in cases of tumors, sclerosis, hereditary or acquired atypical position, and impacted gallstones (Table 1).

Method

The neodymium:aluminum-garnet (Nd:YAG) laser, (type Medilas 2, MBB, Ottobrunn, FRG) with continuous wave mode, 1064 nm (and 1318 nm), and maximum power output 110 W (40 W) was used.

Transmission system was a quartz mono-fiber 0.6 mm in diameter with a Teflon cover, coaxial carbon dioxide flow, and apical metal jet. Diameter of the whole system was 2.0 to 2.6 mm, with transmission of 90 to 100 W (30 to 35 W). Shooting distance from tip to target tissue was 5 mm. The effect of the laser beam is observed through the endoscope using shots of unlimited duration. Olympus sideview fiberendoscope (TJ F 10) with an extra large instrumentation channel, 4.2 mm in diameter was used.

Technique

Tumors

Vaporization or coagulation of indurated malignant structures was carried out with wavelength of 1064 nm and 90 to 100 W using a paintbrush technique, in 2 to 3 sessions, with intervals of 2 to 4 days. The total amount of energy applied depends on tumor structure and size, up to 20,000 J. Coagulation of soft adenoma tissue was attained with 1318 nm. Insertion of a stent was done as soon as the

Table 1   Nd:YAG Laser Treatment of Obstructions of the Duodenal Papilla (from May 1984 to April 1987)

Etiology of the Stenosis	Patients	No	Initial	Sufficient	Excellent
			Success		
Adenoma/adenocarcinoma	7	–	1	4	2
Sclerosis	2	–	–	–	2
Impacted gallstone	2	–	–	–	2
Atypical position	1	–	–	1	–
	12	–	1	5	6

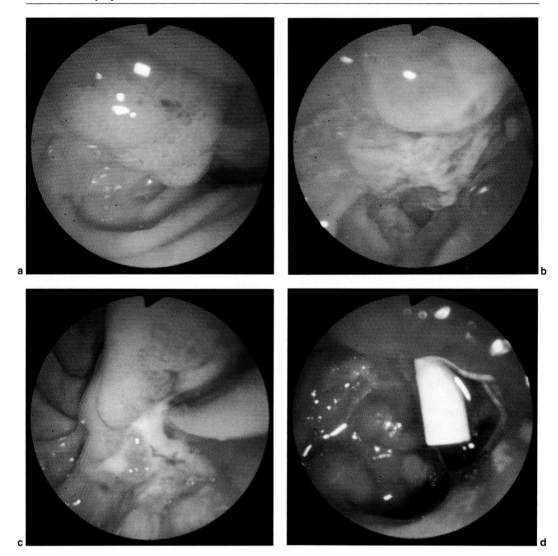

Fig. 1 A 73-year-old woman with penetrating adenocarcinoma of the pancreas with protruding papilla. **a** The ostium cannot be located by endoscopy. **b** After coagulation of the whole visible part of the tumor, the treated tissue is white. **c** Two weeks later, nearly the whole duodenal part of the tumor has vanished. In the depth of a residual ulcer in the region of the papilla, the ostium is intubated. **d** Endoscopic retrograde cholangiography was performed and a stent for biliary drainage was pushed into the regular position.

lumen of the desired duct could be identified. Goals of the treatment included: (1) in cases of duodenal obstruction, palliative recanalization of the duodenum, the common bile duct, and the pancreatic duct; in cases of limited tumor growth, especially in adenomas, destruction of the whole tumor as a complete and possibly curative measure; in all cases repeated treatment and follow-ups are necessary (Fig. **1**).

Sclerosis and Atypical Position

Vaporization with a maximum power of 90 to 100 W (30 to 35 W) starts at the orifice of the papilla 10 to 20 mm in the proximal direction, cutting the wall between the retroduodenal common bile duct and the duodenal lumen following the longitudinal preputial fold. In renarrowing of the ostium after several months, retreatment may be necessary. Energy is up to 2000 J (Fig. **2**).

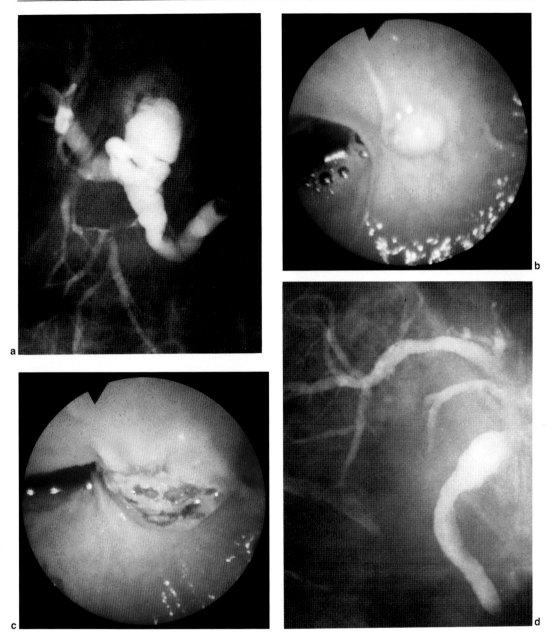

Fig. 2   An 80-year-old male patient after stomach resection (Billroth II). **a** A stone in the common bile duct shown by radiography. **b** The sclerotic papilla in an atypical position cannot be cannulated. **c** Situation immediately after laser coagulation. **d** Success of treatment shown by endoscopic retrograde cholangiography several weeks later.

Impacted Gallstone

The extended mucosa wall close to the stone is incised with maximum power up to 15 mm in the oral direction until the insertion of a basket into the bile duct is possible. Otherwise, step by step cautious laser destruction of the stone can be attempted.

Results

Between May 1984 and April 1987, 12 patients with diseases of the duodenal papilla were treated with the Nd:YAG laser. Five were men, seven were women and the mean age was 73.7 years (range: 56 to 87 years). All had symptoms caused by an obstruction of the biliary and the pancreatic system with retrograde congestion of the secretions, with hyperbilirubinemia, hyperamylasemia, inflammatory signs of cholangitis, pancreatitis, etc. The different indications are shown in Table 1.

In all 6 patients with a malignant tumor, treatment was initially successful. Permanent maintenance of a duodenal passage for the endoscope and the drainage of the bile and the pancreatic secretions into the duodenum was achieved in part by repeated treatments. In two adenocarcinomas (2 and 3 cm in diameter) and the adenoma, a complete local remission was achieved (follow-up, 1 to 2 years). In one patient with a far-advanced tumor, obstruction of the duodenum due to aggressive growth of the tumor made further treatment impossible after a period of 6 weeks.

Each of the two patients with sclerosis of the papilla were only treated once, with complete clinical success. The previous signs of recurrent pancreatitis vanished and had not recurred after a period of 20 to 28 months.

In the case of an 80-year-old man after partial resection of the stomach (Billroth II) with an atypical position of a sclerotic papilla and a calculus in the choledochus, two sessions were necessary to stabilize the primarily successful opening of the papilla with the laser because of a slight tendency to renarrowing 4 weeks after the first session (see Fig. 2).

In the two cases of impacted gallstones, we succeeded in one session in opening up the papilla and fragmenting the stone.

In all patients, no severe complications of the laser treatments were observed. Only the patient who had undergone Billroth II resection developed recurrent cholangitis in intervals of weeks to months after laser papillotomy.

Discussion

The most common and clinically important disorder of the duodenal papilla is obstruction that stops the outflow of bile or juice of the pancreatic gland into the duodenum. When surgery is not indicated because it is not possible or too risky for the patient, various measures are known for a more conservative management of the different types of stenoses. The usual method of treatment is the sphincterotomy with a papillotome using high-frequency diathermy (2). In a small number of patients, it is not possible to insert the papillotome primarily, the complementary cutting catheters or bougies are not sufficient and a percutaneous transhepatic procedure (1) seems not to be advantageous. In those cases of pathologic alteration of the papilla, the Nd:YAG laser is an alternative instrument.

Tumors of the Papilla, Including Neoplasms of the Pancreas and the Biliary Tract Penetrating into the Duodenal Lumen

In such cases, tumor growth can make it impossible to cannulate the ostium of the desired duct. A primary laser coagulation reduces the tumor mass within a few days. In smaller tumors a complete local destruction of the adenoma or adenocarcinoma is induced. Sometimes, the whole sphincter is additionally destroyed. In nearly all cases the ostium of the ducts becomes visible in the depth of the healing ulcer after laser coagulation. If necessary, a prosthesis can be inserted without an additional electrosurgical cut. Although part of a basically palliative concept of treatment, in some patients curative results can be achieved.

Sclerosis

The laser can be used as a precutting instrument by creating a hole that makes it possible to advance the diathermy probe into the choledochus. If the prepapillary part of the common bile duct is prominent and evident under the longitudinal plica, a complete laser sphincterotomy includes the additional advantage of the hemostatic effect of the laser beam.

Atypical Position

This may be hereditary or acquired, i. e., after partial stomach resection. In some of these cases the laser as a noncontact procedure is superior to the electrotomes that have to be manipulated in a distinct direction with contact and a certain pressure in intubating the desired duct, a procedure that cannot always be performed successfully.

Impacted Gallstone

If the papillotome cannot be pushed forward between the gallstone and the extended orifice, laser coagulation and vaporization of both the wall of the ostium and the gallstone can be done with the usual continuous wave Nd:YAG laser. The fragmentation of biliary calculi is necessary in stones of large size. Most of them can be cut and fragmented into smaller parts. Only in the case of material of high consistency is a pulsed laser needed (4).

Summary

The Nd:YAG laser, wavelength $1.06 \mu m$, is an efficient complementary endoscopic therapeutic method in the management of papillary disorders when the usual papillotomes fail. In tumors, complementary laser coagulation is advantageous (6) when compared with electrocautery. Whether the hemostatic effect of laser light is a clinically relevant advantage cannot yet be concluded, but it is conceivable that superior coagulation of tissue and vessels surrounding the cut may lower the risk of bleeding.

References

1. Chen M-F, Jan YY: Percutaneous transhepatic removal of common bile duct and intrahepatic duct stones with a fiberoptic choledochoscope. Gastrointest Endosc 32: 47, 1986
2. Classen M, Demling L: Endoskopische Sphinkterotomie der Papilla Vateri und Steinextraktion aus dem Ductus choledochus. Dtsch Med Wochenschr 99: 496, 1974
3. Kawai K, Nakijima M, Misaki F: Late results of EST in Japan. In: Demling L, Roesch W (eds): Operative Endoskopie. Berlin: Acron Verlag, 1979, 135
4. Lux G, Ell C, Hochberger J, Müller D, Demling L: The first sucessful endoscopic retrograde laser lithotripsy of common bile duct stones in man using a pulsed Nd YAG laser. Endoscopy 18: 144, 1986
5. Sander R, Poesl H: Endoscopic papillotomy with the Nd YAG laser. Endoscopy 17: 1985, 115
6. Sander R, Poesl H: Treatment of benign gastrointestinal tumors with the Nd YAG laser. Endoscopy 18: (Suppl 1): 57, 1986

Lithotripsy of Common Bile Duct Stones

C. Ell, G. Lux, D. Müller, and J. Hochberger

Since the introduction of endoscopic papillotomy (3, 4), and the extension of the technique by the addition of mechanical lithotripsy (6), the endoscopic removal of bile duct stones has been generally accepted, in particular in patients carrying an increased surgical risk. Ninety percent of all stones found in the common bile duct can be removed, retrogradely, via the endoscope. However, hard, very large, or impacted stones still resist endoscopic treatment.

Alternative developments, such as electrohydraulic lithotripsy (12), ultrasound lithotripsy (5), and chemical dissolution of gallstones (1), have not been able to close the remaining gap. The extracorporeal shock wave lithotripsy of common bile duct stones is a new but expensive nonoperative alternative and requires, in addition, sometimes general anesthesia (23).

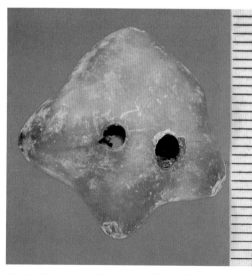

Fig. 1 Thermal melting and drilling effects after cw Nd:YAG energy application (contact. 15 W × 10 s, 150 J).

Experimental Studies and Clinical Applications

Continuous Wave Laser

In 1981, Orii et al. (20) reported the first successful destruction of common bile duct stones with the aid of the neodymium:yttrium-aluminum-garnet (Nd:YAG) continuous wave (cw) laser in man using transcutaneous-transhepatic cholangioscopy. Further reports followed by Orri et al. in 1983 (21), and by Kouzu et al. in 1985 (13, 14). Kouzu et al. pointed out that contact laser lithotripsy with sapphire tips was particularly suitable for the destruction of cholesterol stones. The first in vitro experiments of gallstone lithotripsy with the aid of a cw laser were done and reported by Mills and coworkers (16) in 1983. In our own first experiments in 80 gallstones in vitro we also concentrated on stone destruction by means of the cw laser (7). Various forms of applying energy were investigated (noncontact, contact with naked fiber, contact with interposed sapphire tip – so-called bullet probe). Depending on the method used, the power output varied between 5 and 100 W, the pulse duration between 0.1 and 10 s. It proved possible to destroy or fragment the gallstones to an adequate extent in less than 10% of the investigated stones. In most cases only thermal melting and drilling effects could be observed (Fig. 1). Therefore, and considering the high risk of thermal injuries when working with a cw laser in the bile duct, it has to be stated that the cw Nd:YAG laser is not suited for endoscopic lithotripsy, neither using the noncontact nor the contact technique.

Pulsed Laser Systems

The first reports on attempts to smash stones with a flash lamp pulsed Nd:YAG laser were published by Bown et al. (2). Owing to the lack of any effect, however, they decided to forego any further investigation (25). Contrary to their findings, we succeeded in reliably and reproducibly destroying gallstones with different irradiation parameters in vitro with the aid of a flash lamp pulsed laser, which was already available in an optimal state (LASAG/Switzerland) (8). The energy required for fragmentation was between 10 and 200 J, the pulse duration in the millisecond range, and the pulse energy between 0.15 and 2.5 J. The time required to fragment the stones varied between 2 and 60 s. Hard and cholesterol-rich stones could be destroyed easier than soft or pigmented stones. The lithotriptic effect is of a thermal nature and can be explained by a very localized high vaporization pressure produced within the stone. The laser light is transmitted via a highly flexible quartz fiber with a diameter of 0.2 mm without any appreciable transmission loss, even when the fiber is strongly flexed. This is one prerequisite for endoscopic retrograde lithotripsy by conventional duodenoscopes or choledochoscopes.

After in vitro tests, acute (8) and chronic animal experiments (unpublished data) were carried out in 14 dogs. After laparotomy, duodenotomy, and transduodenal papillotomy, 18 human gallstones were implanted; it was possible to destroy 14 endoscopically by laser light. No acute or chronic complications, such as perforation, cholangitis, or stricture were seen in postmortem radiograms of the common bile duct and in histologic examinations 4 weeks after laser lithotripsy.

Similar lithotriptic effects could also be achieved with flashlamp pulsed tunable dye lasers for wave lengths between 450 and 700 nm (18). In this case, too, a 0.2 mm thin quartz fibre is sufficient for light transmission. Whether the lithotriptic effect is exclusively of thermal or partly of mechanical nature, is, at present, uncertain. There are some experimental data suggesting that the mechanism of stone fragmentation involves a laser-initiated plasma at the stone surface. The plasma absorbs laser light and expands rapidly, generating acoustic waves similar to the Q-switched Nd:YAG system (19). One advantage of the dye laser system might be seen in the fact that gallstones, in particular pigmented stones, absorb more light energy than the surrounding bile duct epithelium, at least in the range of wavelengths used. Therefore, the risk of thermal lesions of the duct might be lower. For pulse energies higher than 30 mJ (maximum 60 mJ), complete fragmentation required fewer than 500 pulses and that means less than 30 J. Pigmented stones could be destroyed with less energy than cholesterol stones. The fragmentation process was not significantly influenced by the pulse duration (0.8 to 360 µs). An important advantage of the dye laser system is the possibility of fragmenting the stones to very small particles of less than 2 mm, which can pass the papilla after papillotomy spontaneously. Recently, the same group reported the fragmentation of gallstones in animals (17), so the first experiences in human beings can be expected in the near future.

First attempts to accomplish lithotripsy of gallstones with the aid of the Q-switched Nd:YAG laser failed because it was not possible to couple high pulse energies into a flexible quartz fiber (16). The advantage of the Q-switched laser system is that thermal injuries of the bile duct do not have to be feared. The use of smaller pulse energies proved to be more effective, but the attempts to break down stones repeatedly resulted in the destruction of the required optomechanical coupling system located at the distal end of the light guide (11). In 1985 we succeeded in coupling high-pulse energies of up to 50 mJ with pulse times in the nanosecond range, in a flexible quartz fiber, and were able to destroy gallstones reliably and reproducibly without causing any damage to the distal focusing facility (10). Recently, Reichel et al. (22) reported on a similar Q-switched laser with a more flexible transmission system due to a different method of inducing the required optical breakdown, namely, using metallic hollow cones – so-called light pipes – at the distal end of the fibre (24). However, to date there are no published reports on animal experiments or clinical experience.

Until now, only our group has been able to gain clinical experience with the endoscopic retrograde laser lithotripsy of common bile duct stones: In May, 1986, we succeeded for the first time in carrying out endoscopic retrograde laser lithotripsy in a human being using a flashlamp pulsed Nd:YAG laser (15) (Fig. 2). By the end of 1987, we had performed laser lithotripsy in nine patients. All of them presented with gallstones that proved to be impossible to remove by conventional endoscopic procedures. In eight of the nine pa-

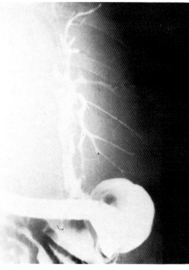
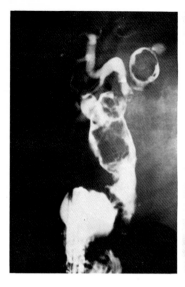

Fig. 2   Laser lithotripsy under direct endoscopic vision; **a** before and **b** after therapy (maximal stone diameter, 4,3 cm).

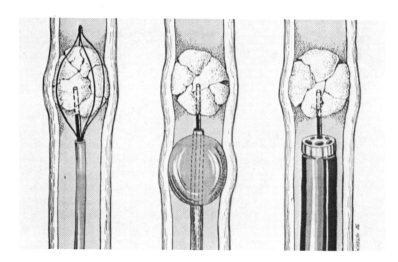

Fig. 3   Variation of the endoscopic techniques used: X-ray control plus lithotriptor-basket or balloon catheter; lithotripsy under direct endoscopic vision.

tients, the stones could be fragmented and in 6 cases removed from the common bile duct; no complications occurred (9). Depending on the anatomic situation, various techniques were used (Fig. 3). In two cases lithotripsy could be performed under direct endoscopic vision. Considering safety, this is the best way to fragment stones without any risk to the bile duct wall. In the near future smaller and more flexible cholangioscopes have to be developed to allow the smashing of the majority of stones under direct endoscopic vision.

As long as lithotripsy has to be performed under X-ray control only, a special attachment is required to ensure a safe distance between the distal end of the light guide and the wall of the bile duct. For very hard stones, which can be caught in a basket, we constructed a laser lithotriptor basket with a central channel for the fiber (Fig. 4). For impacted stones we use a balloon catheter with a central bore for the light guide (Fig. 5).

Even if the first endoscopic retrograde laser lithotripsies in man have been performed

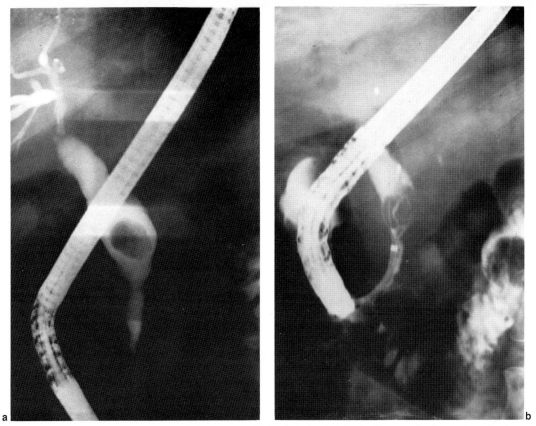

Fig. 4 Laser lithotripsy. **a** X-ray controlled by means of lithotriptor basket; **b** after laser application, a sharp fracture line can be seen (maximal stone diameter, 20 mm).

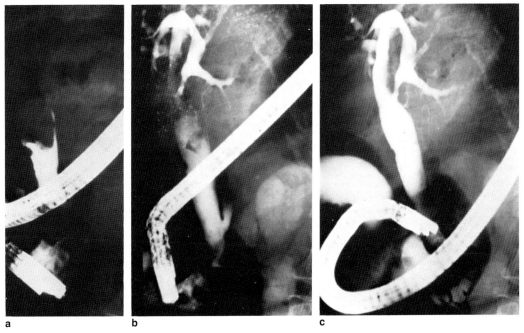

Fig. 5 Laser lithotripsy, X-ray controlled by means of balloon catheter with a central channel for the fiber; **a** before, **b** during, and **c** after therapy (maximal stone diameter, 3.8 cm).

successfully, this method is still in its initial stage. At present, it is not possible to predict which laser system will prove most useful in the clinical application. Further developments and improvements concerning laser systems, energy application, endoscopes, and attachments are necessary to justify the use of laser lithotripsy in daily clinical work with regard to its practicability, cost efficiency, and safety.

References

1. Allen MJ, Borody TJ, Bugliosi T, May GR, LaRusso NF, Thistle JL: Rapid dissolution of gallstones by methyl tert-butyl ether. N Engl J Med 312: 217–220, 1985
2. Bown SG, Mills TN, Watson GN, Swain P, Wickham JE, Salomon PR: Laser fragmentation of biliary calculi. XII. International Congress of Gastroenterology, Lisboa, Portugal, September 16–22, 1984
3. Classen M, Demling L: Endoskopische Sphinkterotomie der Papilla Vateri und Steinextraktion aus dem Ductus choledochus. Dtsch Med. Wochenschr 99: 496, 1974
4. Demling L: Operative Endoskopie. Med Welt 24: 1253, 1973
5. Demling L, Ermert H, Riemann JF, Schmolke J, Heyder N: Lithotripsy in the common bile duct using ultrasound. Endoscopy 15: 226, 1984
6. Demling L, Seuberth K, Riemann JF: A mechanical lithotriptor. Endoscopy 14: 100, 1982
7. Ell C, Hochberger J, Müller D, Giedl J, Lux G, Demling L: Gallensteinlithotripsie mittels Neodym YAG-Dauerstrichlaser. Unpublished data, 1986
8. Ell C, Hochberger J, Müller D, Zirngibl H, Giedl J, Lux G, Demling L: Laserlithotripsy of gallstone by means of a pulsed neodymium YAG-laser in in vitro and animal experiments. Endoscopy 18: 92, 1986
9. Ell C, Lux G, Hochberger J, Müller D, Demling L: Laserlithotripsy of common bile duct stones. Gut. 29: 746–751, 1988
10. Ell C, Wondrazek F, Frank F, Hochberger J, Lux G, Demling L: Laser-induced shockwave lithotripsy of gallstones. Endoscopy 18: 95, 1986
11. Hofmann R, Schütz W: Zerstörung von Harnsteinen durch Laserstrahlung. Experimentelle Grundlagen und in vitro-Versuche. Urologe 23: 181 A, 1984

12. Koch H, Rösch W, Walz V: Endoscopic lithotripsy in the bile duct. Gastrointest Endosc 26: 16, 1980
13. Kouzo T, Sato H: Endoscopic laser treatment of intrahepatic stones. Prog Clin Biol Res 152: 321, 1984
14. Kouzu T, Ymazaki Y, Maruyama M, Murashima M: Cholangioscopic lithotomy using Nd:YAG laser by means of contact-type rod. 2nd Nd: YAG laser conference, München 1985
15. Lux G, Ell C, Hochberger J, Müller D, Demling L: The first successful endoscopic retrograd laser lithotripsy of common bile duct stones in man using a pulsed neodymium YAG laser. Endoscopy 18: 144–145, 1986
16. Mills T, Swain P, Watson G, Bown SG, Salmon PR: Comparison of thermal and photoacoustic fragmentation of biliary calculi using continuous wave and giant pulse lasers. Lasers Surg Med 3: 156, 1983
17. Nishioka NS, Anderson RR: Fagmentation of biliary calculi with tunable dye lasers. Gastrointest Endosc 32: 157, 1986
18. Nishioka NS, Levins PC, Murray SC, Parrish JA, Anderson RR: Fragmentation of biliary calculi with tunable dye laser. Gastroenterology 93: 250, 1987
19. Nishioka NS, Teng P, Deutsch TF, Anderson RR: Mechanism of laser-induced fragmentation of urinary and biliary calculi. Lasers Life Sci 1987 (In press)
20. Orii K, Nakahara A, Takase Y, Ozaki A, Sakita T, Iwasaki Y: Choledocholithotomy by YAG laser with a choledochofiberscope; case reports of two patients. Surgery 90: 120, 1981
21. Orii K, Ozaki A, Takase Y, Iwasaki Y: Lithotomy of intrahepatic and choledochal stones with YAG-laser. Surg Gynecol Obstet 156: 485, 1983
22. Reichel E, Schmidt-Kloiber H, Schöffman H, Dohr G, Hofmann R: Laserinduzierte Stoßwellenlithotripsie (LISL). XVI. Congress of the German Society of Endoscopy, Erlangen, March 20, 21 1987
23. Sauerbruch T, Delius M, Paumgartner G, Holl J, Wess O, Weber W, Hepp W, Brendel W: Fragmentation of gallstones by extracorporeal shock waves. N Engl, J Med 314: 818, 1986
24. Schmidt-Kloiber H, Reichel E, Schöffmann H: Laserinduced Shock Wave Lithotripsy (LISL). Biomed Technik 30: 173, 1985
25. Watson GN, McNicholas TA, Wickham JE: The fragmentation of urinary and biliary calculi. Fourth annual conference on Lasers in Medicine and Surgery. London, January 22, 23 1986

Palliative Therapy of Malignant Tumors

D. Fleischer

Malignant neoplasms of the colon and rectum are common in the United States and Europe. With approximately 140,000 cases annually, colorectal cancer (CRC) is the second most common cause of cancer in the United States (1).If cure of the disease is possible, surgery should be regarded as the treatment of choice in almost all instances. However, in many patients it is recognized at the time of presentation that surgery will not likely be curative but is performed for palliative purposes. Most often, these patients have advanced disease with either extensive local progression or widespread distant metastases. In such patients, the symptoms are often obstruction, bleeding, or diarrhea. It is in this group of patients that endoscopic laser therapy (ELT) may offer an important alternative to surgery and to other modalities. There is also an important role for ELT in the patient in whom CRC presents with large bowel obstruction. The operative mortality in these patients, whether treated by primary resection or staged tumor resection, is high. There is evidence suggesting that ELT for decompression before surgery may reduce morbidity and mortality rates (5, 9).

In this chapter I shall discuss patient selection for ELT for CRC. I shall also review my own technique, pointing out possible alternative approaches by other investigators. Afterward, I shall discuss the results of therapy by a wide variety of experienced endoscopists around the world. Finally, I shall "dust off" my crystal ball and try to project what the future might hold.

Methods

Patient Selection

When determining whether or not a patient who has CRC is a candidate for ELT, I ask three questions:

1. Is the patient a candidate for treatment?
2. What are the goals of treatment?
3. Is ancillary treatment planned?

In determining the patient's candidacy for therapy, I must convince myself that cure by surgery is not possible or that the patient is not a surgical candidate because of his general medical condition. If there is any possibility for cure and there are no medical contraindications to operation, I do not believe that ELT should be performed. I believe that in the future we may reach a stage where our preoperative assessment is such that we can clearly determine the extent of the tumor and know that laser therapy will be curative, but I do not believe that we have as yet reached that stage. As soon as it is clear that a cure is not possible, there are other factors that will help the physician predict whether ELT is likely to be of value. The first of these factors is related to the patient's symptomatology. If the symptoms are bleeding or obstruction, then there is good evidence that ELT may be of benefit. However, if the patient's main symptoms are pain, then, in my experience, ELT will not be useful, since this is presumably related to disease outside of the colonic lumen. The second set of factors relates to the geography of the tumor. For esophageal cancer, these parameters have been clearly defined (7). Although the same study has not been carried out for

CRC, I do believe that it is likely to be more effective when the tumor is exophytic rather than submucosal, when it involves a straight segment of the colon rather than a sharp bend, and when it represents a short segment rather than a longer one.

The second question that I like to clarify in my own mind, and of course with the patient and referring physician, is what the goals of treatment should be. Potential benefits and risks must clearly be defined before treatment. The patient must be told that the intended laser treatment is not curative and the recurrent symptoms are likely to develop. The patient must understand that it is likely that subsequent palliative endoscopic treatments will be required in a few months. With a better understanding of what is to be expected, the patient is much more tolerant of all the different aspects of therapy.

Third, I always like to determine in advance whether or not ancillary treatment is planned. For example, if I am opening up an obstructed colonic lumen immediately before surgery, then decompression is the only goal, and one need not destroy as much tumor as one would if that were the only treatment. Although there is not an unanimous opinion as to whether or not radiation therapy or chemotherapy have a role for CRC, if these therapies are to be carried out, it is best to consult with the other physicians to determine the sequence of therapy.

The next issue to be considered before laser therapy is full definition of the tumor geography and its extent. With the exception of the patient who is treated on an emergency basis, I always obtain three tests before laser therapy. These are:

1. Barium enema
2. Screening endoscopy
3. Imaging study

The purpose of the barium enema is to define the path and configuration of the colonic tumor. I want to know how sharp the angulations are in the colon and what is the degree of narrowing. I also will observe for complications of the tumor, such as perforation, and it is useful to define this before endoscopic therapy. Although I do not believe that this test is absolutely essential, I find it useful both in planning treatment and comparing the pre-ELT status to the post-ELT situation. In the patient in whom significant obstruction is an issue, the radiologist must be adivised to be careful about advancing barium proximal to the obstruction.

Endoscopic assessment of the tumor is mandatory. Although this may be carried out at the same time that the first treatment will be administered, the endoscopist must have a feel for the geography of the tumor. As mentioned previously, I like to know if it is exophytic, how sharp the angulations are, and how friable the tumor is. When the tumor is hemorrhagic, then a great deal of smoke is likely to develop, with thermal injury from the laser, and this will make the treatment more tedious.

An imaging study provides additional information. Most of my personal experience is with computed tomography (CT) scans, but we are just beginning to use magnetic resonance imaging and endoscopic ultrasonography (EUS). I believe that the latter technique will be extremely valuable. The work of Tytgat has shown that this is extremely sensitive for staging tumors of the esophagus. He also believes that EUS is the most accurate device for staging rectal cancer (14). It allows for clear visualization of the extent of intramural infiltration and the adjacent perirectal lymph node involvement. Rectal cancer is usually visualized as a hypoechoic intramural lesion. Early rectal carcinoma can be suspected when a circumscribed lesion limited to the mucosal and submucosal layers is found. Since we are just beginning to use EUS at Georgetown, my main experience is with CT scans of the rectal area. One is attempting to obtain the same information as discussed with EUS.

Preparation

The preparation before the procedure is generally as follows. It is usually performed as an outpatient procedure. If a patient has symptoms of obstruction or profuse bleeding, then hospitalization is required. Before the procedure, bowel cleansing is performed. If there are lesions in the rectum, enemas may suffice. Generally, I prepare the patient with an oral electrolyte solution (Golytely or Colyte). Usually 4 to 5 liters is given in the evening before the procedure. After bowel preparation, good visualization is more likely and the chance of an explosion is reduced.

The procedure is routinely carried out in the endoscopy suite, except on rare occasions when the tumor is close to the anorectal verge and epidural anesthesia is required. Otherwise, I routinely sedate the patient with meperidene and midazolam intravenously. The patient is routinely positioned in the left lateral decubitus position. In cases in which treatment of the anorectal area is involved, a lithotomy position may provide better access.

My own work has been carried out with a neodymium:yttrium-aluminum-garnet (Nd:YAG) laser with power output of 1 to 100 W. I have used the 1.06 μm wave length. Others have used the argon, carbon dioxide, or 1.32 Nd:YAG laser. When the lesion is close to the anus, there appears to be a definite advantage to using the argon laser, which causes less pain with treatment. When I have used the YAG laser in these circumstances, I have had to either inject a local anesthetic or use epidural anesthesia.

My largest experience is with the standard noncontact fibers, although on some occasions I have used the contact fiber or used a naked fiber, which is inserted into the tumor directly. A wide variety of endoscopes should be available. Most commonly, I use the endoscopes of standard caliber. However, in cases of obstruction it may be necessary to use the smaller diameter endoscope. When using flexible instruments, I now use a video system almost exclusively. In addition to its superb resolution, I find it to be an extreme advantage to view the procedure on a video monitor. This allows my assistant to know exactly what I am doing and to be more helpful during the procedure. An additional benefit is the fact that safety glasses, which I find to be quite a nuisance, are usually not required with videoendoscopy. At least on some occasions, for anorectal tumors, an anoscope or special therapeutic proctoscope, has an advantage.

Most of the accessories that are used for the procedure are standard; however, when dealing with patients with obstructions, dilations may be required before the procedure. In such instances, balloon dilation with or without a guidewire may be required, or an over-the-wire polyvinyl tapered dilator could be used. These will be discussed in more detail in the following section.

Technique

I will describe technique as it relates to both treatment for obstruction and bleeding (15). It will also be necessary to differentiate between tumors in the anorectal area from those in the more proximal colon.

For the patient with CRC in whom the primary problem is hematochezia or occult blood loss, the goal of therapy is cessation of hemorrhage and reduction of tumor size. In such instances, I try to coagulate the tumors, so I use a power setting in the range of 70 to 80 W with pulse durations of 0.5 s with a noncontact probe. I try to place the laser fiber approximately 1 cm from the tumor and treat as much of the tumor surface as possible. If there is blood on the surface during the treatment, it invariably will vaporize and become black, but in areas of the tumor that did not have blood on the surface, the white coagulative effects are seen. Generally, the goals of therapy can be accomplished with one to two treatments, although subsequent treatment may be required as tumor sloughs and a new hemorrhagic surface presents.

For the patient who has obstruction that is not in the anorectal area, my treatment technique is as follows. I advance the endoscope to the distal end of the tumor. It is hoped that the endoscope will be able to pass through the entire tumor so that the geography will be fully defined. I will have gotten some idea from the barium enema or imaging study about the length and anatomy of the tumor. If the endoscope can pass from the distal margin to the proximal margin, I find that valuable for assessing the tumor. There is some debate as to whether or not treatment should begin at the more distal or proximal margin; the answer is not clear-cut. It is always best to get a full view of the entire tumor length before beginning treatment. However, after I have done that in some patients, I will begin the treatment at the most proximal margin (i.e., after I have advanced from the distal margin through the tumor to its most proximal point, and then to the normal lumen). On some occasions, I begin with the distal margin. There is some debate as to whether or not the goals of treatment should be vaporization or coagulation. I find in most cases that I treat, that both thermal effects are achieved. My own preference is to vaporize the tumor, since more tumor will be destroyed and I believe that this reduces the total number of treatments that are required. To accomplish this, I use powers of 80 to 90 W with a pulse duration of 2 s or longer. I am looking for changes of vaporization, which is noted by a divot that forms where the beam strikes the tumor. If I begin the treatment at the most proximal edge, I will withdraw it and treat as I come back to the most distal end of the tumor. In treating, I am looking for areas where obstruction is likely to cause symptoms. I am not trying to obtain a cosmetically perfect effect. The treatment session will end when I have treated a maximal amount of tumor.

Sapphire tips can be adapted to conventional fibers so that treatment can be carried out. With the contact method, powers of 15 to 20 W are used and the fiber tip is in direct contact with the tumor. In my experience this has been far more tedious than noncontact methods, but in some situations it has the advantage of being able to reach around corners and, by using the side of the contact probe, to treat areas that would be difficult to reach with the conventional fiber. It should be emphasized that this is not a situation of one approach versus the other, and in any given case I may use both approaches.

What do I do when the endoscope advances to the distal margin of the tumor and it will not pass (Fig. 1)? The endoscopist has several options in this situation. One approach is to switch to a smaller caliber endoscope. Alternatively, treatment can be begun at the distal margin using either the standard noncontact probe or the contact probe. More often, however, I attempt to dilate the constriction so that I can define the whole anatomy before beginning treatment. This may be accomplished with either a through-the-scope balloon dilator, a toposcopic thru-lumen everting catheter, or by passing a guide wire.

Dilation before laser therapy with a guide wire is demonstrated in Figure 2. The endoscope is advanced to the distal margin of the tumor. The guide wire is passed through the tumor and the endoscope is removed. Over the guide wire, a tapered polyvinyl dilator (shown here) or balloon dilator is passed. After dilation, the endoscope can be advanced through the obstruction and treatment can be begun at the proximal end of the tumor if this is desired.

Anorectal cancer presents specific problems, and I find that the most diffucult area to

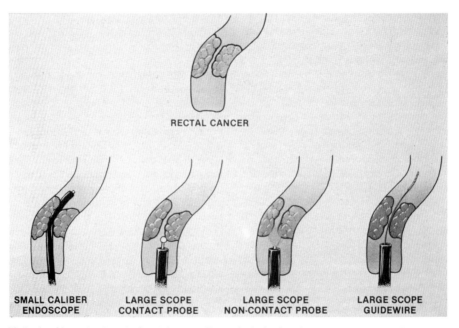

RECTAL CANCER

| SMALL CALIBER ENDOSCOPE | LARGE SCOPE CONTACT PROBE | LARGE SCOPE NON-CONTACT PROBE | LARGE SCOPE GUIDEWIRE |

Fig. 1   Methods of laser treatment of rectal cancer if standard-sized endoscope cannot pass through obstructed lumen.

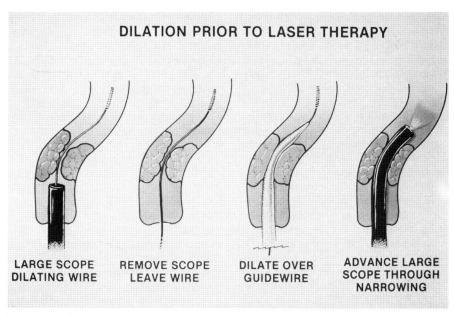

DILATION PRIOR TO LASER THERAPY

LARGE SCOPE   REMOVE SCOPE   DILATE OVER   ADVANCE LARGE
DILATING WIRE   LEAVE WIRE   GUIDEWIRE   SCOPE THROUGH
                                                               NARROWING

Fig. **2**   Method of dilating obstructed colorectal cancer to allow passage of endoscope.

treat. Also, in my experience, the results are less good. For the patient who has an anorectal tumor that is causing obstruction or bleeding or in the situation of a villous adenoma that is being treated because the patient is a nonoperative candidate or an abdominoperineal resection is believed to be undesirable, therapy will be carried out. In some cases treatment can be carried out with an endviewing endoscope in a noncontact probe or via an anoscope. However, often complete treatment is not possible and other methods are required. These are demonstrated in Figure **3**. One approach is to use the turnaround view with a flexible endoscope. This works well for a tumor that is not close to the endoscope itself, but one must be careful when performing a turnaround view that the beam does not strike the endoscope, because this can lead to instrument damage with leakage.

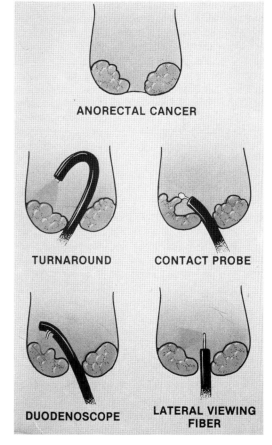

ANORECTAL CANCER

TURNAROUND   CONTACT PROBE

DUODENOSCOPE   LATERAL VIEWING
                    FIBER

Fig. **3**   Different treatment techniques for use of ▶ laser for anorectal cancer.

Another approach is to use the contact probe. Because laser energy emits from the side of the probe as well as tip, access may be achieved that could not be achieved with the end-aiming, noncontact probe. Alternatively, a conventional duodenoscope can be used that allows for side-aiming. Recently, I have had some experiences with the lateral aiming fiber developed by Hashimoto (8). On some occasions, a flexible instrument is not perfectly suited and I have used a hand-help probe that can be delivered through an anoscope or a rectal dilator.

After treatment, diet is advanced based on the patient's condition until solid foods can be tolerated. A stool softener or bulk laxative is generally prescribed. If a second treatment is required, the patient will generally be kept on a liquid diet until the next treatment. If the patient is in the hospital, the second treatment is generally carried out in 48 hours. For outpatients, the second treatment can be carried out 5 to 7 days later.

The patient is warned that with tissue edema on some occasions obstructive symptoms may be temporarily worse rather than better, although this is far less common with colonic tumors than with esophageal tumors. On some occasions, pain medication is required. If the goals of treatment are accomplished after one session, then follow-up treatment is usually carried out in approximately 6 weeks, or whenever symptoms recur.

Results Therapy

The largest experience for a laser usage for patients with CRC is by Lambert (10). Between 1981 and 1986, he treated 449 patients in Lyon. The lesion was located in the rectum in 322 patients (72%). Advanced cancer was present in 357 patients (80%). Cancer foci and adenomatous polyps were the therapeutic indication in the other 92 patients (20%).

Lambert usually used an Nd:YAG laser emitting 1.06 nm. He uses it both with a co-axial gas flow and a standard fiber or with a bare fiber; in the latter situation the beam is defocused, allowing interaction with the tissue. He varies the power from 40 to 100 W, depending on the topography of the lesion. On some occasions, he uses the Nd:YAG laser emitting 1.32 nm powers of 20 to 25 W. He finds that this is most useful for new neoplastic lesions and those located in the lower rectum.

He uses carbon dioxide laser for the source for destruction of neoplastic lesions in the low rectum. He believes that the carbon dioxide laser generates less pain than the YAG laser.

The most common indication for laser photodestruction by Lambert is palliation of acvanced cancer. He uses laser therapy in the symptomatic patient who is considered to be a poor operative risk because of old age or associated disease, liver metastases, or extensive regional invasion. He initiates tumor destruction at an initial setting and chronic maintenance treatments carried out at intervals of 8 to 12 weeks. He does not believe that its use in the colon proximal to the sigmoid is generally appropriate. Best results are obtained in exophytic, noncircumferential tumors. When the tumor is ulcerative, poor results are usually obtained and circumferential stenosis may be a complication.

Lambert also uses the laser for curative treatment in colorectal cancer, when the tumor is of small size (not more than 3 cm), exophytic, nonulcerated, without deep infiltration of the intestinal wall, and when the tumor is well-differentiated. Usually, this is used when the tumor is in the lower rectum. Lambert also uses the laser for curative treatment of colorectal adenoma with cancer foci. In about 10% of the cases, resection of colorectal adenoma with the diathermic snare is not possible. In such patients, foci of cancer may be demonstrated. When laser therapy is carried out in this group of patients, close follow-up is warranted.

The results of palliative treatment of sigmoid carcinoma by laser therapy was recently reported by Brunetaud et al (3). They reported on 95 patients who underwent endoscopic outpatient laser therapy for palliation, using either Nd:YAG or argon laser at the Lille Laser Center. All patients were classified as inoperable because of coincidental medical conditions or the extent of the tumor. They divided the patients into two groups: ten patients in group 1 had exophytic tumors of less than 3 cm in diameter, and 85 patients in group 2 had more advanced tumors. Local control of tumor was obtained in all but one patient without complication, and 85% of group 2 patients were symptomatically improved by the treatment. The survival rate (by life-table analysis method) at 24 months was only 19%, but the precentage of surviving patients who remained symptomatically improved was high (90% at 3 months to 68% at 24 months). Factors influencing improvement of survival rates include the main symptom at the beginning of treatment, the reason for choosing laser treatment, and circumferential extent of tumor base. There was one fatal perforation and one perirectal abscess. The investigators concluded that laser photocoagultion was able to control small rectosigmoid carcinomas if the patient is unable to undergo incisional surgery. Laser treatment provided relief of symptoms in an operable patient with advanced rectosigmoid carcinomas.

Mathus-Vliegen and Tytgat (12) reported on their own experience with the usefulness and safety of laser photocoagulation in 63 patients with colorectal cancer. The laser was evaluated in the treatment of 16 patients with obstruction, 32 patients with bleeding, 15 patients with combined symptoms. Luminal patency could be restored in 15 patients (94%); hemostasis was achieved in 23 patients (72%); and treatment was effective in 13 of 15 patients (87%) in whom the tumor caused both bleeding and obstruction. In the 56 evaluable and initially responding patients, no beneficial long-term results were achieved in six patients, because major complications occurred. In three patients, post-treatment hemorrhage requiring blood transfusion occurred; and in one patient a perirectal abscess was present; the latter was responsible for the only probably treatment-related death. Transient stenosis and laser-induced bleeding as minor complications were present in 19%. The beneficial effect of laser photocoagulation was generally present after 2 to 3 sessions. Forty-six patients could be discharged from the hospital and the treatment could be continued for them as outpatients. Further hospital admission was avoided in 39 patients. The investigators concluded that the laser treatment for palliation of obstructing or bleeding colorectal cancer proved to be efficacious, safe, and rapidly effective, and that it could be considered a valuable alternative to more conventional surgical intervention in many patients.

The use of preoperative Nd:YAG laser treatment of obstructive colon cancer is reported by Kiefhaber et al. (9). Laser recanalization was carried out on 57 patients with obstructive colonic carcinoma, and in 54 patients (95%) successful treatment was accomplished. The investigators had undertaken this approach because morbidity and mortality rates with staged operations for colon cancer are still high. They presumed that if preoperative recanalization could be achieved by laser vaporization, then symptoms of ileus could be resolved, which would permit preoperative peroral bowel lavage. By performing preoperative laser treatments, the mortality was reduced to 8.8%, which is considerably lower than the result when preoperative laser treatment is not carried out. Similar results were obtained by Eckhauser (4) in much smaller series in the United States. Bown et al. (2) reported the results in 17 patients with cancer of the rectum or distal sigmoid who were considered inoperable. Using the YAG laser for symptoms of rectal bleeding, obstruction, diarrhea, or incontinence, significant improvement was achieved in 15 patients (88%) (2). No complications were reported. The investigators emphasized that this technique is the only nonsurgical therapy that can be used safely for lesions above the perineal flexion and provides palliation in these seriously ill patients.

A study by Mellow (13) adresses not only the medical aspects of the ELT for rectal cancer, but also considers some economic aspects of treatment. He calculated the cost for 21 patients undergoing ELT for rectal cancer and compared it with the cost of 35 patients undergoing surgery. The total cost for surgical treatment (i. e., physician's fees, all hospital charges) was $ 22,000. The total cost for laser treatment patients was $ 4600. Since laser therapy requires repeated treatments throughout the patient's life, the total lifetime costs were calculated for ten patients with known metastatic disease at the time of presentation. The total cost was $ 8500 in this group of patients, significantly less than that of surgery.

Discussion

The results of ELT for palliation in patients with tumors of the lower gastrointestinal tract are encouraging. The data must be viewed with the perspective that these were reported by very experienced endoscopists and it is not clear whether or not these results can be obtained by a less experienced physician. It should also be underscored that there are no controlled studies comparing ELT with other modes of treatment.

Having said that, it should also be stated that the initial results demonstrate the possibilities for successful outcome by this treatment. As new technologies are more refined, it is hoped that even more effective treatment can be carried out and complications can be reduced. It is also emphasized that ELT should not be viewed as being in competition with surgical treatment. It is definitely not an "either/or situation." The important study by Kiefhaber et al. (9) demonstrated that best results for the patient are obtained when there was good cooperation between the endoscopist and the surgeon.

In my own view, one can set guidelines as to when it is appropriate to use the laser and when it should not be used. If cure is possible with surgical treatment, and abdominoperineal (AP) resection is not required, I believe that ELT has no role. It also has little place in most patients with rectal tumors even if AP resection is required, but that cure is an expected outcome. It also has no role in treating patients in whom the endoscopic characteristcs are not favorable (i. e., the tumor is submucosal or extremely ulcerated).

On the other hand, I think laser treatment has a definite role as a potential curative therapy in some small cancers when the patient is inoperable. I think it should also be used in most patients in whom an AP resection would be required for palliation.

Whereas the latter two categories seem to be reasonably clear to me, I think the exact role of laser therapy in certain situations is not fully defined. In the patient who has a small tumor, in whom it is believed that laser therapy could be curative, I do not believe that we have reached the degree of sophistication with our current preoperative staging to know that laser treatment is as effective as surgical resection. It is also unclear to me what the best management is for the patient with CRC who is an excellent operative candidate but in whom there is evidence of extensive local disease or in whom there are liver metastases. Further data will be required to clarify the best approach in the latter group of patients.

Outlook for the Future

It was not too long ago that the standard treatment for any colonic polyp was exploratory laparatomy with surgical resection. To-day, for the large majority of polyps, that treatment would be considered inappropriate and outdated. We now have endoscopic access to the entire colon, and most polyps that are either pedunculated or small and sessile can be removed by snare using electrocoagulation. In a recent editorial that I wrote, I emphasized that snare polypectomy for a pedunculated colon polyp represents the perfect treatment (6). By analyzing the characteristics that make that treatment ideal, it is possible to map out the future with regard to endoscopic laser therapy for malignant tumors of the colon.

Characteristics that portend successful endoscopic laser therapy are: (1) pathologic process that is discrete from normal tissue; (2) good access to the pathologic process; (3) a method for delivering treatment; (4) a way of assessing the entire pathologic process; and (5) an insurance that complete removal or destruction of the lesion has occurred.

Often, the endoscopic appearance of CRC is such that the endoscopist does not even know the surface boundaries of the tumor. Certainly, he does not understand the depth of invasion. The situation is very different than with the pedunculated colon polyp, where boundaries are very clear. Solutions to the problem are possible by using substances such as hematoporphyrins that are selectively localized in neoplastic tissue. It may be possible to define borders better than can be done today. I have already mentioned the work with EUS, which may provide precise definition of both the lateral margins and submucosal extent of the tumor. Finally, it may be that videoendoscopy can also allow us to define the edges and borders better than can be done with current instruments. By using the combination of computer analysis in association with videoendoscopy, it is probable that more information can be gleaned.

Access to the entire tumor for ELT is not always ideal. In the future, some of the newer small caliber endoscopes will allow the passage through even the most narrow lumen. Smart endoscope (robotic) instruments, which are self-advancing and lumen seeking may also be of value. Holographic instruments may also have a role in the future. There is also room for the development of new types of fibers. In a short time, alternatives to the conventional end-aiming, noncontact probes, interstitial treatment fibers, and lateral aiming fibers.

Further generations of these fibers and newer ones may help the endoscopist gain better access and destruction of the lesion. It is also possible that fibers carrying lasers of other wavelengths may have utility in this situation.

We currently are dependent on biopsy or operative samples for a definition of tumor histologic characteristics. It is well recognized that endoscopic biopsies taken from the surface of the tumor at specific points may not be representative of the entire tumor. In the future, I believe that histologic definition may be obtained without tissue sampling. It may be that computer-generated information from videoendoscopes and from EUS will allow us to define histologic characteristics without a tissue specimen. It is also possible that information gleaned from biopsies will tell us more about the tumor than just its mere histologic features. The antigenic properties of surface markers as well as chemical information may be useful in determining how a specific neoplasm may respond to laser treatment and even in defining the best wavelength for therapy. Certainly, if ELT is to replace surgery for colon cancer, the endoscopist must have information that allows him to know that the entire pathologic process has been treated. The advantage of surgery is that it puts the entire colon cancer in a jar in a pathology laboratory and the surgeon can sleep well at night knowing that the entire process has been removed. The endoscopist will need similar certainties if he is also to sleep well. At the present time, ELT for malignant tumors is primarily palliative. Until now, that is the way that it should be. It is hoped, however, that future technologic advances will allow endoscopic therapy to be a primary one and that conventional surgery will only be used in the exceptional situation. Although that may sound a bit unlikely, it must be remembered that one-quarter of a century ago, colon polyps were handled in a similar fashion. Great strides have been made with ELT for colonic neoplasms and the future is bright.

References

1. American Cancer Society: Cancer Statistics, 1986. CA. 36: 9, 1986
2. Bown JG, Barr H, Matthewson K, Swain CP, Clark CG, Boulos PB. Brit J Surg 73: 949, 1986
3. Brunetaud JM, Manoury V, Ducrotte P, Cacheland D, Cantor A, Paris JC: Palliative treatment of rectosigmoid carcinoma by laser endoscopic photoablation. Gastroenterology 92: 663, 1987
4. Eckhauser ML: Endoscopic laser vaporization of obstructing left colonic cancer to avoid decompressive colonostomy. Gastrointest Endosc 33: 105, 1987
5. Fielding LP, Stewart-Brown S, Blesovsky L: Large bowel obstruction caused by cancer: A prospective study. Brit. Med J 2: 515, 1979
6. Fleischer D: Laser and colon polyps. Technology and pathology: The courtship continues. Gastroenterology 90: 2024, 1986
7. Fleischer D, Sivak MV: Endoscopic Nd:YAG laser therapy as palliation for esophagogastric cancer. Parameters affecting initial outcome. Gastroenterology 89: 827, 1985
8. Hashimoto D: The development of lateral laser radiation probes. Gastrointest Endosc 33: 240, 1987
9. Kiefhaber P, Kiefhaber K, Huber F: Preoperative neodymium:YAG laser treatment of obstructive colon cancer. Endoscopy 18: 44, 1986
10. Lambert R: Laser in colorectal cancer. Presented at International Symposium on Endoscopic Therapy of Gastrointestinal Bleeding and Neoplasms, Washington, D.C., Georgtown University: April 4, 1986, p 204
11. Mathus-Vliegen EMH, Tytgat GNJ: Laser ablation and palliation in colorectal malignancy: Results of a multicentre inquiry. Gastrointest Endosc 32: 939, 1986
12. Mathus-Vliegen EMH, Tytgat GNJ: Laser photocoagulation in the palliation of colorectal malignancies. Cancer 57: 2212, 1986
13. Mellow MH: Endoscopic laser treatment in colorectal cancer. Presented at Digestive Disease Week. Chicago: ASGE National Course, May, 1987
14. Tio TL, Tytgat GNJ: Atlas of transintestinal ultrasonography. Rijswijk, The Netherlands, Smith Kline and French, 1986 (p 23)
15. Waye, J, Geenan J, Fleischer D: Techniques of therapeutic endoscopy. Philadelphia Saunders, 1987 (p 31)

Colorectal Adenomas

E. M. H. Mathus-Vliegen and G. N. J. Tytgat

The laser, being a relatively recent treatment device in gastroenterology, has entered an important and crucial phase after one of disbelief and scepticism and after a period of uncritical and unlimited belief and confidence in the efficacy, usefulness, and safety of the method. Nowadays, guidelines for application have to be determined and indications and contraindications have to be defined. The potentials and advantages on the one hand, but also the limitations and drawbacks on the other, have to be delineated. This applies to both main treatment fields: a. that of hemostasis in acute and potentialy bleeding lesions and b. that of tumor irradiation for cure in benign and early stage malignant lesions and for palliation in cancers.

In hemostasis, some controversy still exists among gastroenterologists about the type of laser that has to be used (4, 9, 10). However, in tumor ablation there is much less disagreement; the neodymium:yttrium-aluminum-garnet (Nd:YAG) laser is proposed for the treatment of massive bulky lesions, whereas the argon laser, if available, is preferred in superficial and small lesions (2, 3, 5, 7). Now surgeons and gastroenterologists appear to be at odds. Consensus exists about the use of laser photocoagulation in the palliation of bleeding and obstructing digestive cancers and both agree on the treatment of benign or premalignant polypoid lesions in certain circumstances. Most of the discussions focus on the decision-making. Surgeons are concerned about two facts: firstly, that a patient is too easily considered inoperable and thereby is condemned to only palliative procedures for cancer, and secondly, that the progress that has been made in transsacral, transsphincteric, and transanal polyp resection and mucosectomy (1, 6, 8, 14, 15, 21) even without general anesthesia, has not yet fully been appraised. In doubtful and incomplete polyp removal by endoscopic polypectomy and certainly in severe dysplasia, focal and even invasive carcinoma, laser treatment and surgery have to be balanced against each other, taking into account the medicosurgical condition of the patient.

In November 1979 we started a prospective trial in patients with colorectal adenoma and in patients with rectal stump polyps after colectomy and ileorectal anastomosis in familial polyposis. The aims were twofold: to investigate the efficacy and safety of laser photocoagulation in the treatment of colorectal adenomas and to study the gross and histologic effects on the colon on both short- and long-term laser photocoagulation. The completeness of tumor ablation, initially achieved in 72%, and the high recurrence rate thereafter, resulting in definite eradication in only 54% at the completion of the analysis, was somewhat disappointing (11, 19). Also, the rate of major complications (stenosis, perforation and post-treatment hemorrhage), although not requiring surgery, in 7% and of minor complications without a need for hospital admission in 24% was unexpected, as were the ten instances (15%) of carcinoma present or developing in the laser-induced ulcer base.

However, three facts were encouraging: the rapid and efficient control of symptoms caused by the adenoma, the easy treatment of multiple polyps in familial polyposis, and the scarless mucosal healing on both short- and long-term therapy. In an attempt to find an explanation for the failures and complications, we carried out a detailed analysis of the patient material (12, 16). From this analysis, it became obvious that the rate of recurrences and complications paralleled the size of the adenoma without relationship to the duration of the treatment period or the amount of energy applied. There was probably some correlation with histologic changes because failures were mainly observed in villous-type lesions. Dysplasia did not influence the results. However, difficult accessibility and problems with aiming of the laser beam were encountered more frequently in extensive lesions, whereas bleeding occurring during laser application occasionally interfered with adequate further treatment. Laser-induced ulceration and edema delayed further treatment. Proper interpretation of the endoscopic appearance after laser application was also a source of problems in that differentiation between remaining adenomatous tissue and healing regenerating epithelium was sometimes difficult.

Based on our initial experience, we were able to define a subgroup of patients for whom laser treatment would be truely useful, i. e., the patients with smaller polyps with severe dysplasia or even focal carcinoma, those with recurrent rectal stump polyps after ileorectal anastomosis in familial polyposis, and those with larger polyps in whom symptoms are troublesome and debilitating.

Meanwhile, gaining more experience also by the treatment of malignant (17, 19) and of potentially bleeding lesions (20), we continued our prospective study. The recently updated results form the basis of this communication.

Patients and Methods

In the period from November 1979 until February 1987, 180 patients entered the study and were divided into two groups. Group 1 included 150 patients with persisting adenomatous tissue after conventional endoscopic polyp removal or with recurrent adenoma after surgical intervention. Information about histologic changes had to be present. The remaining nonpedunculated and flat tissue could not be removed by polypectomy and patients were unsuitable for surgery because of serious medical illnesses or unfavorable anatomy of the lesion. Some patients refused operation.

The adenomas were classified into large (extensive), intermediate, and limited (small) growth using the following criteria: (1) extensive adenomas (n = 60) involving at least two-thirds of the circumference or extended longitudinally over at least 4 cm; (2) intermediate adenomas (n = 56) between 1 and 4 cm in extension or with an insertion base over less than two thirds of the circumference; (3) a small lesion (n = 34) consisting either of residual polypoid tissue or stalk after snare

polypectomy or of small flat, nonpedunculated islands of adenomatous tissue with a diameter of at least 1 cm. Another prerequisite was the presence of severe dysplasia or even focal carcinoma.

For analysis, adequate long-term follow-up of more than 20 weeks was required. Eradication of adenomatous tissue was considered to be complete only after normal findings at endoscopy and multiple negative biopsies, obtained over a period of at least 12 weeks. In contrast to our previous study, those patients who were referred for the treatment of the adenoma, but who presented with a cancer during follow-up, are not included in the analysis. These patients will be considered separately.

Since complete, histologically proved eradication may be an unrealistic aim in extensive, tapestry-like lesions in the elderly, patients with persisting neoplastic tissue despite treatment were also analyzed according to the amount of remaining tissue and to the timing of the observed endoscopic reduction and symptomatic relief.

Group 2 consisted of 30 patients with familial polyposis coli treated during follow-up of recurrent polyps in the rectal stump after subtotal colectomy and ileorectal anastomosis. A 6-month interval was indicated for the surveillance of the rectal stump: however, more frequent surveillance (at intervals of 1 to 3 months) was indicated if multiple polyps or recurrences or a combination of the two were present. The development of adenocarcinoma, the occurrence of villous or dysplastic changes in polyps or flat mucosa, and uncontrollable growth and multiplication of polyps were considered as an indication for surgical intervention.

Methods

Treatment Technique

In patients with adenomas, primary treatment consisted of snare polypectomy, with piecemeal debulking in massive lesions and with tenting up and providing a pseudopeduncle in smaller sessile polyps. If further debulking proved to be impossible, laser therapy was started after an interval of 2 to 3 weeks, which allowed for healing of the coagulated area. Pulses of 1.0 s at maximum output (usually 70 to 80 W calibrated at the tip) were applied in large sessile lesions; in tiny and superficial lesions and in patients with rectal stump polyps a pulse duration of 0.5 s with 45 to 70 W was used. In addition, an overlap in heat conduction was avoided by providing an interspace between the hit points in a stippling fashion and by timing the interval between two pulses. The length of each session was determined by the quantity of energy applied and by the endoscopic appearance of the lesion. White discoloration due to protein denaturation was pursued. Black discoloration and smoke formation had to be avoided but were sometimes inevitable in a blood-covered lesion. In circumferential growth, only half the lesion (or sometimes even less) was treated at the first session. In longitudinal spread, treatment was given to the entire adenoma from proximal to distal, but limited to one-quarter of the circumference. The laser light was aimed at the lesion tangentially, more or less parallel to the luminal axis. Only in bleeding spots perpendicular targeting first around and thereafter at the center of the bleeding spot was carried out.

Patients were prepared in the outpatient department with a sodium phosphate enema. Only patients with proximally located lesions required a large tap water enema. No premedication or antispasmodic agents were used.

Technical Data

An Nd:YAG laser (Medilas MBB, Messerschmitt, Bölkow and Blohm, Munich, FRG: power 100 W, pulse duration 0.1 to 9.9 s) was connected to a water-cooling circuit (distilled water 10 l/min; 3.5 bar). The invisible infrared laser light was transmitted by a quartz fiber encapsulated in a Teflon sheath with a Helium-Neon, visible red laser as the aiming beam. The preset pulse duration was controlled by a foot switch, and the output at the tip was calibrated and adjusted before each session. Coaxial carbon dioxide needed for cooling and cleaning of the fiber tip and of the area under treatment was delivered at a flow rate of 0.8 L/min. Overdistension of the bowel was prevented by a rectal cannula, introduced along the endoscope to allow the free escape of gas. Treatment was usually carried out with the flexible TCF-1S Olympus sigmoidoscope with a large (5 mm diameter) instrumentation channel and with the CF-1TI or LB-3W Olympus colonoscope with washing facilities to clean the area under treatment.

Results

Group 1

In a series of 150 consecutive patients with colorectal adenoma, 115 patients could be analyzed, seven patients refused further treatment, and in 14 patients, the time lapse required for adequate treatment or assessment of eradication was too short. Cancer was detected during the course of the treatment in one small, in seven intermediate and in six extensive adenomas. The latter patients were analyzed separately.

Patients with Extensive Growths

Of 60 patients, 47 could be analyzed (Tables **1–4**, Fig. **1**). Cardiovascular (9), pulmonary

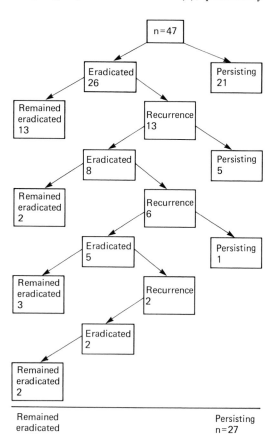

Fig. **1** Overall cumulative results in extensive adenoma.

Table **1**   Results of the First Treatment Period in Adenomas*

	Extensive Adenoma (n = 47)	Intermediate-Sized Adenoma (n = 39)	Small-Sized Adenoma (n = 29)
Age (yr)	72 (42–93)	70 (35–86)	70 (38–96)
Follow up (wk)	120 (20–361)	112 (22–337)	109 (22–302)
Eradicated	26	33	28
Sessions (no)	8 (2–19)	4 (1–13)	2 (1–4)
Period (wk)	43 (6–137)	25 (4–69)	11 (2–69)
Energy (J)	27 835 (4145–135 849)	12 280 (840–47 389)	2572 (350–12 320)
Not eradicated/Persistent	21	6	1
Sessions (no)	14 (5–41)	8 (2–12)	2
Period (wk)	101 (24–361)	66 (24–128)	28
Energy (J)	54 641 (19 698–97 069)	17 458 (2298–38 379)	3039

* Numbers are given as means and the range is given in parentheses.

Table **2**   Complications of Laser Coagulation

	Extensive Adenoma (n = 47)	Intermediate Adenoma (n = 39)	Small Adenoma (n = 29)	Polyposis (n = 25)
Major complications*	3	3	–	1
Stenosis	2	–	–	–
Post treatment hemorrhage	0	3	–	1
Serositis	1	–	–	–
Minor complications	27	12	4	3
Asymptomatic, transient stenosis	5	3	1	–
Minor post treatment hemorrhage	11	8	3	1
Laser-induced hemorrhage	1	–	–	–
Serositis	2	–	–	–
Pain	8	1	–	2

* Necessitating hospital admission, endoscopic or surgical intervention.

Table **3**   Conditions Interfering with Adequate Laser Treatment

	Extensive Adenoma	Intermediate Adenoma	Small Adenoma	Polyposis
Pain during treatment	15×	4×	–	–
Difficult accessibility	14×	7×	3×	–
Retraction/convergence of folds/ asymptomatic transient stenosis	12×	7×	5×	–
Ulceration	6×	3×	–	–
Friability and hemorrhage	3×	3×	–	–
Fecal flow	5×	5×	–	–

Table **4**   Parameters Associated with Treatment Resistance and with Stenosis in Different Polyp Sizes

	Extensive Adenoma	Intermediate Adenoma	Small Adenoma
Characteristics of resistant adenomas V/TV/T*	10/10/1	2/3/1	0/0/1
Circumference			
> 3/4	8	–	–
< 3/4, > 1/2	6	–	–
< 1/2	7	3	–
Length (cm)	7	2	–
Stenosis			
Treatment (no)	7 (3–14)	3	3
Period (wk)	40 (12–101)	11 (5–18)	13
Energy (J)	30 779 (8441–86 510)	9915 (3500–15 190)	4550

* Histology: villous (V); tubulovillous (TV); tubular (T)

(5), and cerebrovascular disease (1), hematologic disturbances (1), diabetes (1), age (2), and miscellaneous conditions (4) precluded surgical intervention. Unfavorable anatomic location, usually requiring major surgery, contributed to a conservative approach in 24 patients. Five lesions were located in the sigmoid, one in the splenic flexure, and 18 in the upper third of the rectum. Surgical resection preceded this treatment in five, surgical polyp removal in eight, complicated by one perforation and three strictures.

Prior endoscopic polypectomy in 34 was complicated in two instances by hemorrhage, once by perforation and once by stricture formation. Histologic investigation revealed tubulovillous adenoma in 25, villous tissue in 19, and tubular adenoma in three. Eleven of the 47 polyps contained severe dysplasia and four focal carcinoma.

Of the 47 patients, 24 were clinically symptomatic. Excessive mucous discharge was noted in 18, diarrhea in 13, hematochezia in ten, abdominal cramps, mild ileus, and fecal incontinence each in three and hypokalemia in one patient. Relief of symptoms was seen in all but one patient, who complained of persistent diarrhea and incontinence, despite considerable reduction in tumor volume. Symptomatic relief occurred after a mean of two treatments, given over 6 weeks, whereas tumor reduction by 75% took much longer: a mean of four treatments over a 16-week period.

All neoplastic tissue could be eradicated in 26 patients after a mean of eight laser treatments administered over 43 weeks. Almost twice as many treatment sessions and treatment weeks did not result in complete ablation in 21. Only residual nests were present in 18 of these 21 patients after 13 treatments over 95 weeks; the three patients who still had considerable amounts of adenoma at endoscopy received 15 treatments over 136 weeks. Follow-up lasted for a mean of 120 (range 20 to 361) weeks. This period was characterized (Fig. **1**) by frequent endoscopic visible recurrences, followed either by repeated eradication or by further persistence of adenomatous tissue after re-treatment. The outcome is illustrated in Figure **1**: 20 of 47 patients were finally free of endoscopic detectable and histologically demonstrable neoplastic tissue. The other 27 continued laser irradiation.

Major complications (see Table **2**) occurred in three patients: symptomatic stenosis in two, which necessitated endoscopic dilatation once and a colostomy in another patient, who had been treated previously by monopolar electrocoagulation over the last 10 years, before resorting to laser treatment. Abdominal pain, thought to be due to serosal irritation ("serositis"), probably caused by transmural necrosis necessitated only one hospital admission, but subsided on conservative treatment.

Minor complications were seen in 27 patients. Asymptomatic transient stenosis was defined as a short segment of narrowed lumen, resistant to the introduction of a large, 13 mm diameter endoscope and often visible as a fibrotic ring, and occurred in five patients.

Treatment was temporary discontinued, whereupon the stenosis resolved spontaneously. Minor post-treatment hemorrhages were seen between days 2 and 11 and on the average occurred at day 7. One laser-induced hemorrhage reacted favorably with continued laser application. In seven of the eight patients who complained of pain in the following days, fever was also present.

Conditions interfering with adequacy of treatment and probably contributing to failures and complications were also analyzed (see Table **3**): especially difficult access to the lesion, partly caused by retraction and stenosis, was a common problem, whereas ulceration and friability occasionally interfered with adequate treatment. In the 21 persistent adenomas, villous and tubulovillous type tissue were equally present (Table **4**). However, an extensive longitudinal spread and extension over the whole circumference occurred obviously more frequently in combination.

Patients with Intermediate Growth

Of 55 patients, 39 could be included in the analysis. Old age (5), surgical complications (4), digestive (4) and hematologic (4) disorders, and cardiovascular (2) and pulmonary diseases (2) made them less suitable for surgery (Tables **1–4**, Fig. **2**). Unfavorably localized lesions were present in 21: five in the sigmoid, one in the descending, one in the transverse colon, one at the cecal floor, with 13 adenomas in the upper third of the rectum. Previous resection had been performed in eight patients and surgical polyp removal in five, complicated by one bleeding, one stricture, and two instances of fecal incontinence. Once, bleeding occurred in 29 patients with prior endoscopic polypectomy. The nature of the neoplastic growth was tubulovillous in 19, villous in 14, and tubular in six. Severe dysplasia was seen in nine, with focal malignancy in four. Symptomatic relief was noted in all 15 patients presenting with hematochezia (12), mucous discharge (5), diarrhea (3), incontinence (1), and abdominal cramping (1) after three treatments given over 7 weeks. As can be seen in Table **1**, tumor ablation was achieved in 33 patients after a mean of four treatments in 25 weeks. In six patients, twice as many treatment sessions did not result in eradication, leaving behind, however, only minute islands of adenomatous tissue. The fol-

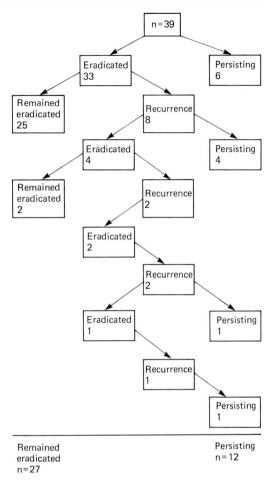

Fig. **2** Overall cumulative results in intermediate adenoma.

low-up period of the intermediate adenoma (mean 112 weeks; range 22 to 337 weeks) was also characterized by recurrences and re-treatments (Figure **2**), with ultimately healing in 27. Major complications (see Table **2**) consisted of three late hemorrhages, with a need for blood transfusion in two and effective laser hemostasis in one. Minor complications occurred in 12 and consisted mainly of asymptomatic stenosis and minor post-treatment hemorrhages, which occurred between days 1 and 10, but as a rule at day 7.

Difficult accessibility because of fibrosis and retraction interfered with adequate therapy. Pain during treatment occurred less often. Histologic changes or extension of the lesion (Table **4**) seemed not to be an explanation for treatment resistance.

Patients with Small Growths

In this group, the data of 29 of 34 patients could be analyzed (Table **1–4**, Fig. **3**). Surgical intervention for these small lesions was not considered appropriate, despite severe dysplasia in 12 and focal carcinoma in two of the 14 villous, 11 tubulovillous and four tubular adenomas. Besides, cardiovascular disease (5), pulmonary insufficiency (1), hematologic disorder (1), and diabetes (1) were present. One resection and two surgical polypectomies already preceded the present treatment; endoscopic polypectomy had been carried out in 25 and was complicated by four hemorrhages. Symptoms were usually absent and relief, therefore, not evaluable.

All tumors except one disappeared on two treatments given over 11 weeks. Recurrences were rare. Permanent eradication was obtained in 28 of the 29 adenomas (Fig. **3**). Also, complications were infrequent; once a stenosis did not require endoscopic dilatation (see Table **2**).

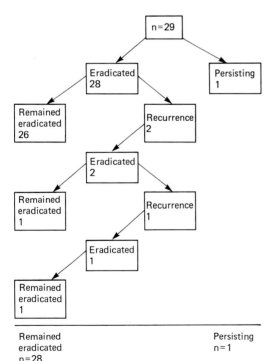

Fig. **3**   Overall cumulative results in small adenoma.

Group 2

Thirty patients of young age (mean 28; range 10 to 64 years) were evaluated during the surveillance of the rectal stump after ileorectal anastomosis. Follow-up data of 25 patients could be analyzed.

In a mean follow-up period of 162 weeks (range 3 to 312), a mean of ten polyps (range 1 to 68) was treated at intervals of 24 weeks (range 1 to 132) with one major and one minor instance of bleeding (see Table **2**). One malignancy in a noncompliant patient was detected. In four a rectal resection with a pelvic pouch and ileoanal anastomosis was performed.

Patients with Malignant Degeneration

In the three subgroups of adenomas, malignancy was discovered during treatment in one small adenoma, in seven intermediate, and in six extensive adenomas. Prior surgical or endoscopic polypectomy specimens were available in 13 of the 14 cases, and on revision none, except for one doubtful exception, had shown malignancy. In only three had prior dysplasia been present, villous tissue was present in ten, tubulovillous and tubular adenoma each in two. In the intermediate form, an ulcer persisted for a mean of 17 weeks (range 6 to 30) after a total of four treatments (range 2 to 9) over 22 weeks (range 4 to 61) when the malignancy was detected on biopsy; while in the extensive form, the persistence of ulceration together with stenosis or convergence of folds was found after 17 treatments (range 9 to 35) given over a period of 75 weeks (range 32 to 99).

A 75-year-old patient from the small adenoma group appeared to have Dukes' C at operation. Four of the seven patients (mean age 60 years; range 35 to 74) in the intermediate group were operated on, and a Dukes' A and Dukes' B carcinoma was found in one and three patients, respectively. Three refused surgery, one is lost to follow-up, one is still alive for 141 and the other for 210 weeks since the start of the treatment. Four of the six with a mean age of 80 years (range 65 to 92) in the extensive adenoma group underwent surgery (one Dukes' A, one Dukes' B, two Dukes' D). Two patients refused surgery, one is lost to follow-up and one has survived for 235 weeks after the start of the treatment.

Discussion

We were at first somewhat discouraged by our own rather mediocre results (19), which contrasted with the excellent results reported by others. However, we decided to continue our prospective study, once we realized that especially the extensive type of adenoma present in 40% in our study group was not included in other series (5, 13, 22). For example, the extensive adenoma group was only present in 19% in Brunetaud et al. (5) series. Since our first reports (16, 19), the patient material has doubled. Initial eradication in the total group of 115 patients was found in 76%, which declined ultimately to 65% because of recurrence of adenomatous tissue.

However, these recurrences appeared to be manageable and remained responsive to laser photocoagulation, an observation that contrasts now with our previous impression (19) that a recurrence was more resistant to therapy. Initial eradication was obtained in 55, 85, and 97% of the extensive, intermediate, and small lesions, respectively. The respective percentages of definite tumor ablation at the end of our study with an appreciable mean follow-up of 114 weeks, are 43, 69, and 97%.

It is important to notice that complete, permanent eradication was difficult, especially in a subgroup of very extensive lesions with an extension over the whole circumference, together with considerable longitudinal spread. Impressive, however, was the immediate relief of symptoms in the usually elderly patient, most of the time bothered by frequent diarrhea, excessive mucous discharge, and incontinence.

In familial polyposis the repetitive treatment of multiple small adenomas was easy and efficient. Healing of the mucosa occurred without nodular deformity, retraction, or scarring.

The overall complication rate of 5% for major and of 33% for minor events is acceptable. There was no mortality. Some important points have to be mentioned here. Post-treatment hemorrhage occurred preferably around day 7. Stenosis (Table **4**) seemed not related to the number of treatments, the total amount of energy delivered, or the histologic type of the lesion. It certainly interfered with further adequate treatment due to difficult access to the lesion, concealed between or behind folds in the shortened, retracted segment or behind fibrotic rings. Ulceration was of importance in two ways. On the one hand, it impeded effective treatment because of intense reflection of laser light by the whitish slough and because of prolongation of the interval period necessary between the treatment sessions. On the other hand, the persistence of ulceration with little healing tendency and even more if it appeared in combination with stenosis, retraction, and outgrowth of the polyp, always raised suspicion of malignant degeneration. Unexplained is our finding that the malignancy was only discovered in the base of the insertion site of the polyp and not in the material removed by polypectomy.

Based on these results and data of morbidity and complication rate, we feel confident in selecting patients as appropriate candidates for laser destruction. Firstly, the treatment is indicated in old patients with troublesome symptoms of adenomatous lesions who are considered less suitable for surgery due to medical conditions or to unfavorable anatomic localization in the upper third of the rectum and higher where only major surgery is the alternative. Preferably, small and intermediate lesions have to be present. In the most unfavorable subgroup of both extended circumferential and longitudinal growth, one has to weigh the burden of the treatment and the predictably less favorable response against the severity and rapid disappearance of symptoms and the risk of non complete and non curative tumor eradication.

Secondly, in patients with rectal stump polyps after ileorectal anastomosis in familial polyposis, regular control and treatment is safe and easy without scarring. However, uncontrollable growth, dysplastic or villous changes in polyps or flat mucosa, and, of course, adenocarcinoma are strict indications for surgical resection.

References

1. Adair HM, Everett WG: Villous and tubulovillous adenomas of the large bowel. J Roy Coll Surg Edinb 28: 318–323, 1983
2. Bowers J: Laser therapy of colonic neoplasms. In: Fleischer D, Jensen D, Bright Asare P (eds): Therapeutic Laser Endoscopy in Gastrointestinal Disease. Nijhoff, Boston 1983 (pp. 139–150)
3. Bown SG: Tumor therapy with the Nd:YAG laser. In: Joffe SN, Muckerheide MC, Goldman L (eds):

Neodymium Yag Laser in Medicine and Surgery. Elsevier, New York 1983 (pp 52–58)

4. Brunetaud JM, Jensen DM: Current status of argon laser hemostasis of bleeding ulcers. Endoscopy 18 (Suppl 2): 40–45, 1986

5. Brunetaud JM, Mosquet L, Houcke M, Scopelliti JA, Rance FA, Cortot A, Paris JC: Villous adenomas of the rectum. Results of endoscopic treatment with argon and neodymium: Yag lasers. Gastroenterology 89: 832–837, 1985

6. Buess G, Theiss G, Günther M, Hutterer F, Pichlmaier H: Endoscopic surgery in the rectum. Endoscopy 17: 31–35, 1985

7. Dixon JA, Burt RW, Rotering RH, McCloskey DW: Endoscopic argon laser photocoagulation of small sessile colonic polyps. Gastrointest Endosc 28: 162–165, 1982

8. Fasano JJ: Surgery of villous tumours of the colon and the rectum. Ann Gastroenterol Hepatol (Paris) 20: 315–323, 1984

9. Fleischer D: Endoscopic therapy of upper gastrointestinal bleeding in humans. Gastroenterology 90: 217–234, 1986

10. Fleischer D: Laser photocoagulation for upper gastrointestinal bleeding: The American experience. Endoscopy 18 (Suppl 2): 52–55, 1986

11. Fleischer D: Lasers and colon polyps. Technology and Pathology: The courtship continues. (Editorial) Gastroenterology 90: 2024–2025, 1986

12. Johnston J: Complications of endoscopic laser therapy. In: Fleischer D, Jensen D, Bright Asare P (eds): Therapeutic Laser Endoscopy in Gastrointestinal Disease. Nijhoff, Boston 1983 (pp 173–185)

13. Löffler A, Dienst C, Velasco SB: International survey of laser therapy in benign gastrointestinal tumors. Endoscopy 18 (Suppl 1): 62–65, 1986

14. Malafosse M, Roge P: Surgical management of villous tumors of the colon and rectum. Dig Surg. 1: 168–171, 1984

15. Mason AY: Surgical access to the rectum, a transsphincteric exposure. Proc Roy Soc Med. 63: 91–94, 1970

16. Mathus-Vliegen EMH: Complications and pitfalls of lasertherapy. Endoscopy 18 (Suppl 1): 69–72, 1986

17. Mathus-Vliegen EMH, Tytgat GNJ: Laser photocoagulation in the palliative treatment of upper digestive tract tumors. Cancer 57: 396–399, 1986

18. Mathus-Vliegen EMH, Tytgat GNJ: Laser photocoagulation in the palliation of colorectal malignancies. Cancer 57: 2212–2216, 1986

19. Mathus-Vliegen EMH, Tytgat GNJ: Nd:YAG laser photocoagulation in colorectal adenoma. Evaluation of its safety, usefulness and efficacy. Gastroenterology 90: 1865–1873, 1986

20. Mathus-Vliegen EMH, Tytgat GNJ: Nd:YAG laser photocoagulation in mucosal vascular abnormalities: A critical analysis (Abstr.) Third congress of ELA (European Laser Association), Amsterdam, November 6–8, 1986

21. Parks AG, Stuart AE: The management of villous tumours of the large bowel. Br J Surg 60: 688–695, 1973

22. Sander R, Poesl H: Treatment of benign gastrointestinal tumors with the Neodymium: Yag laser. Endoscopy 18 (Suppl 1): 57–79, 1986

Benign Stenoses

J. F. Riemann

Advantages of photocoagulation with the aid of the laser, such as the avoidance of direct contact with the tissue, control of the thermal reaction, and avoidance of an electric current passing through the tissue, are the reasons for the expansion of the indication spectrum for laser. It is, therefore, not surprising that attempts have also been made to use laser therapy to treat benign stenoses of the lower gastrointestinal tract, too (1, 4, 7,9). This may be especially the case in patients with deeply located gastrointestinal tract strictures caused by the end-to-end anastomosis (EEA) autosuture stapling procedure (2).

Patients and Method

In the period between April 1, 1985 and June 30, 1987, we used the laser beam to treat seven patients presenting with benign stenoses of the lower gastrointestinal tract. Four of the patients presented with scar strictures after a prior resection of the bowel for either carcinoma or endometriosis; in three of the patients the stenosis was due to inflammatory bowel processes (Crohn's disease) without any signs of active Crohn's disease.

For therapeutic colonoscopy, we made use of both gastroscopes and colonoscopes (XQ 10, CF-IBW). As a rule, the patients were premedicated with pethidin 100 mg, and N-butylscopolammonium bromide, 2 ml. In two patients in whom the initial treatment with the laser proved very painful, the procedure was repeated under peridural anesthesia.

Our technical approach was as follows: In the first session, quadrant incisions were made; in the same session, dilation of the stricture with the aid of a balloon catheter was attempted (Figs. **1–3**). At the second session,

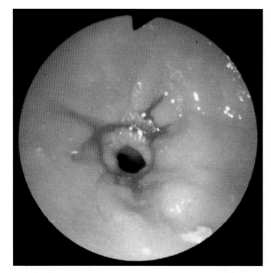

Fig. **1** High-grade stricture in the rectum after deep anterior resection and end-to-end anastomosis using stapler.

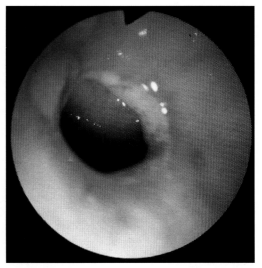

Fig. **2** Condition after the first laser session.

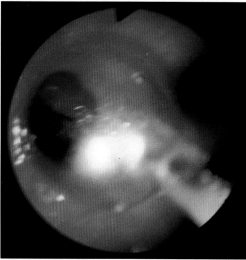

Fig. **3**   Ballon dilation.

Table **1**   Laser Therapy of Benign Strictures of the Lower Gastrointestinal Tract

Patient Data	Postoperative Strictures	Crohn's Disease
Patients	4	3
Location (Rectosigmoid/Colon)	3/1	3/0
Succes rate	3/4	3
Number of Sessions	2 (1–3)	2 (1–3)
Free intervals (months)	4 (1–8)	3 (2–10)
Follow-up (months)	20 (10–26)	18 (12–24)
Recurrence rate	2–4	2/3
Complications	–	–
Surgery	1/4	–

held 2 to 3 days later, an attempt was made to pass the thin caliber, subsequently the thick caliber, endoscope through the stenosis. The objective was considered to have been achieved when a conventional colonoscope (diameter, 1.8 cm) readily passed through the stenosis (Fig. **4**).

Results

The results achieved are shown in Table **1**. In six of seven patients, passage through the stenosis was fully reestablished. As a rule, this required two to three sessions with the laser. No complications were observed. The patients with cicatricial strictures experienced pain dur-

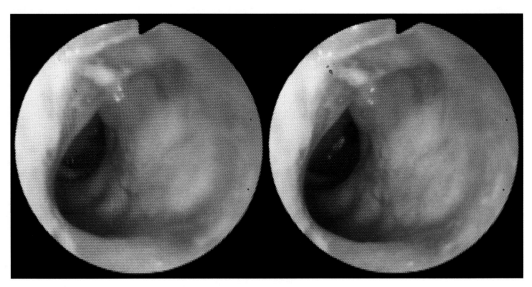

Fig. **4**   Result after two laser treatments with fairly complete recanalization.

ing treatment with the laser, for the most part complaining of a sensation of heat. As was to be expected, no reactions were observed under peridural anesthesia, and in these patients the results were, owing to the elimination of the pain reaction, better. In a follow-up period of 20 months, recurrences occurred in four of seven patients in the period between 3 and 4 months, each of which was successfully re-treated in the manner described. Meanwhile, one patient had to be operated on after 1 year of treatment due to a high recurrence rate at short intervals.

Case History

In a 42-year-old female patient, a colectomy with ileorectostomy was carried out for Crohn's disease, 1 year before her first admission to our department. The anastomosis was located 10 cm above the anal canal. Postoperatively, a vascular complication of the iliac artery that required the use of a vascular prosthesis occurred. The patient presented with a filiform stenosis and the clinical symptoms of subileus. Using the combination of laser therapy and dilation with the balloon catheter as already described, complete dilation of the stricture was accomplished in two sessions. At present, the patient has follow-up examinations at 4 month intervals. Under this treatment, there has been no flare-up of Crohn's disease.

Discussion

The treatment of choice for strictures of the lower gastrointestinal tract, in particular after prior surgical interventions, is definitive surgical correction. In a number of cases, however, vaporization with the laser is available as a possible alternative. This is especially the case

when the strictures are very low, thus making them readily accessible to endoscopic treatment. The EEA stapling technique is widely used in colorectal, intestinal, and esophageal surgery for creation of EEA, end-to-side, and side-to-end anastomoses (2). Despite the fact that a stricture of this origin is rare at this moment, one may face the problem of increasing numbers due to increasing use of the procedure.

Electrocautery or bougienage of these strictures is not very effective (4). However, a satisfactory dilation can be accomplished with extensive laser vaporization, aided by dilation with the balloon catheter. At the present time, an apparent disadvantage is the relatively high incidence of recurrent stenosis. However, these recurrent lesions are amenable to treatment in the same manner. It is possible that the tendency to recur is associated with an initially inadequate depth of the incision. With increasing experience, and in particular when pain is excluded by peridural anesthesia, results have been improved by performing an additional incision with the laser. It is worth noting that all our patients were referred to us for laser treatment by surgical departments. This also applies to the three patients with Crohn's disease stenoses, who were asymptomatic with regard to the underlying disease. The main symptoms in the case of low stenoses were those of subileus. Immediately after laser therapy, symptoms were absent in all of the patients. Two of the seven patients reported pain on defecation for several days after the procedure. Our results are in agreement with those indicated in a survey (Table 2), which revealed good to excellent results in 65.4%, satisfactory results in 11.5%, and poor results in 23.1% of the cases. Over an average follow-up period of 11 months, the recurrence rate was also 40% (6).

Table 2 Laser Therapy of Benign Strictures of the Lower Gastrointestinal Tract

	Good	Satisfactory	Poor
Results	34 (65.4%)	6 (11.5%)	12 (23.1%)
Location	Rectosigmoid 33/52 Colon 19/52		
Follow-up	1–26 months (mean 10)		
Recurrence rate	21/52 (40.4%)		
Complications	1/52 (1.9%) ⟶ Perforation		

Löffler et al. (3) also reported on an international survey of laser therapy in benign gastrointestinal tumors and stenoses, including 27 patients with either rectosigmoid (22 patients) or colon (5 patients) stenoses. Their results were in most cases excellent, except for one patient in whom the long-term results were disappointing.

According to Tytgat (11), the results are better when the stenosis is relatively short and are less than optimal in cases of long stenotic lesions. The combination either with bougienage or ballon dilation may well improve the immediate and the long-term results.

Laser therapy of scar stenoses in the lower gastrointestinal tract is both possible and likely to be successful in selected cases; it should be carried out in close cooperation with the surgeon, after careful weighing of alternative procedures and the risks involved.

References

1. Chen P-C, Wu C-S, Chang-Chien C-S, Liaw Y-F: YAG laser endoscopic treatment of an esophageal and sigmoid stricture after end-to-end anastomosis stapling. Gastrointest Endosc 30: 258, 1984

2. Cutait D E, Cutait R, Silva JH, et al: Stapled anastomosis in colorectal surgery. Dis Colon Rectum 24: 155, 1981

3. Löffler A, Dienst C, Velasco SB: International survey of laser therapy in benign gastrointestinal tumors and stenoses. Endoscopy 18 (Suppl 1): 62, 1986

4. Nagao F (ed): Endoscopic Treatment in the Digestive Tract. Asakura Shoten, Tokyo 1983 (p 115)

5. Riemann JF: Lasertherapie im Gastrointestinaltrakt. Internist Prax 26: 645, 1986

6. Riemann JF: Laser-therapy of the lower GI-tract. Symposium on the laser in gastroenterology with emphasis on upper GI-malignancies. World Congress of Gastroenterology, Sao Paulo, Brasil, September 12, 1986

7. Riemann JF, Kohler B: Behandlung mit Laserstrahlen im Verdauungstrakt. Fortschr Med 27–28: 525, 1986

8. Sander R, Poesl H: Endoskopische Lasertherapie. Leber Magen Darm 6: 234, 1985

9. Sander R, Poesl H: Treatment of non-neoplastic stenoses with the neodymium-YAG-laser. Indications and limitations. Endoscopy 18: 53, 1986

10. Sasako M, Iwasaki Y, Takami, et al: Endoscopic laser treatment for the post-operative anastomotic stricture of the digestive tract. Gastroenterol Endosc 24: 2028, 1982

11. Tytgat GNJ: Benign stenoses – benign tumors. Endoscopy 18 (Suppl 1): 60, 1986

Photodynamic Therapy

Basic Principles

S. G. Bown

Photodynamic therapy (PDT) has attracted a lot of interest in the last few years as a new technique with the potential for localization (by fluorescence) and selective destruction of malignant tumors (particularly small, multifocal lesions). It is based on the systemic administration of certain sensitizing drugs, which are retained with some selectivity in tumors and can be activated by light to produce a local cytotoxic effect. Undoubtedly, local tumor destruction by this method is possible, although for comparable light doses, the extent of tissue damage in tumors is very little more than in adjacent normal tissue. The real value of PDT will probably lie more in the nature of the biologic effects produced, since these are different from thermal damage. Tumors seem to melt away, whereas normal areas heal with regeneration. However, many of the factors involved are poorly understood, and it is too early to be sure what role PDT will play in the treatment of human disease. This chapter will outline the current state of knowledge of PDT in gastroenterology, with particular emphasis on experimental work that has tried to establish the nature of photodynamic damage to normal and tumor tissue.

Background

The first attempts at PDT date back to 1903, when Tappenier and Jesionek (30) used eosin and fluorescein in combination with light to treat skin carcinomas, although the results are not clear from the available literature. Most work since has focused on porphyrin derivatives as the photosensitizing agents. The first report of porphyrin fluorescence in tumors came when Policard (25) in 1924 observed red fluorescence from experimental animal sarcomas exposed to light. This was probably due to the accumulation of endogenous porphyrins, but Auler and Banzer (1) injected porphyrins into tumor-bearing animals and demonstrated tumor fluorescence and a subsequent toxic effect on illumination.

Hematoporphyrin is difficult to obtain in a pure form, and it was in attempts to do this that Lipson et al. (22) in 1961 arrived at a new product that had superior properties with respect to tumor localization. This was produced from the action of sulfuric acid and acetic acid on hematoporphyrin and has become known as hematoporphyrin derivative (HPD). HPD and dihematoporphyrin ether/ester (DHE; thought to contain a higher percentage of the active ingredient or ingredients of HPD), are both incompletely defined mixtures of porphyrins, but are the most studied and currently the most frequently used drugs for work on fluorescence visualization and selective destruction of tumors with light (16). However, new groups of drugs with similar biologic properties, but which are much easier to handle chemically, are now being studied, particularly the phthalocyanines (27).

Tissue damage by PDT is thought to involve the production of singlet oxygen (33). After its systemic (usually intravenous) administration, the sensitizing agent can be activated by light of a wavelength matched to one of its absorption peaks. This activated form can elevate oxygen from its ground state (triplet oxygen) to the much more reactive singlet state. Singlet oxygen is short lived and can produce a toxic effect (most likely on the cell membrane, although probably also on other cellular organelles) in the region of the cell where it is formed.

Photosensitizer

It is often thought that the key to tumor destruction with PDT is the selective retention of the sensitizing agent in malignant neoplasms. It is now clear that, with the exception of intracranial tumors (34), this is a relatively minor factor, and the final biologic effect may depend more on the distribution of the applied therapeutic light and the local response of the target area (normal or neoplastic) to a particular level of absorbed light energy and singlet oxygen production. However, selective retention is the factor that has been used to characterize the technique, and so will be considered first.

Early work showed that selective fluorescence could be excited in about 75% of malignant tumors in man after systemic administration of HPD (18). Subsequent studies revealed that the level of fluorescence correlated poorly with absolute concentrations of HPD (measured by radioactive labeling) (17), and there are no detailed studies comparing fluorescence intensities with absolute HPD concentrations for tumors and the normal organs in which those tumors arose. There are several excellent studies comparing the fluorescence of neoplastic areas, particularly carcinoma in situ, with the surrounding normal tissue in the bladder (5) and bronchi (15).

The factors determining the distribution of HPD in different organs are complex and poorly understood. The highest concentration is found in liver, slightly less in kidney and spleen, with much lower levels in muscle and skin. The highest level in most normal organs in mice is reached within 3 to 6 hours of a bolus dose, and decreases slowly after 2 to 3 days. Levels in a mouse mammary carcinoma have been shown to follow a similar pattern and to be in the middle of the range of values seen in normal tissues (17). However, measurements of total HPD concentration such as this do not explain the selective fluorescence that is seen in tumors. Indeed, in humans, when one would expect the retention of HPD to be slower, selective fluorescence can be seen in areas of carcinoma in situ in resected bladders only 2 to 3 hours after administration (5). In the original article (18) maximum tumor fluorescence was seen after 3 hours, which had disappeared by about 18 hours. This has yet to be explained.

Bugelski et al. (9) proposed that in normal tissues the rapid clearance of extravasated serum proteins precludes the establishment of an equilibrium condition between serum protein and cellular binding sites for HPD, whereas the relatively leaky vessels and the known lack of a competent lymphatic system in tumors permit trapping of serum proteins in the extracellular fluid, thus permitting an equilibrium to be established between HPD bound to serum proteins and that bound to cellular binding sites (9). They also showed the importance of the tumor vasculature. Using autoradiography, they found that the concentration of HPD is up to five times greater in the vascular stroma of tumors than in or around individual malignant cells. The localization of sensitizer in vascular stroma was reflected in observations after exposure of sensitized tumors to light. The first effects were seen on the blood vessels which became narrowed with sluggish blood flow, to be followed by extravasation of red cells (28). There is no immediate effect on malignant cells. Indeed, if small subcutaneous tumors in mice are treated with HPD and light at dose levels known to eradicate the tumor if left in situ, but tumor cells are removed and transplanted immediately after exposure to light, they grow normally in culture (19). This is strong confirmatory evidence that the tumor cells die secondary to failure of their blood supply. The importance of the vascular effect has also been shown in normal rat jejunum (26). Undoubtedly, there is a toxic effect on individual malignant cells, which has been shown in tissue culture experiments, but the light dose required is higher, and there is no major difference between normal and malignant cell lines (10).

HPD is far from the ideal sensitizer. It is an ill-defined mixture of porphyrins whose action is not well understood, with relatively weak tumor selectivity. Also, it has only a weak absorption peak in the red part of the spectrum (at about 630 nm), where light penetration of tissue is best, stronger peaks occurring at shorter wavelengths in the near ultraviolet, blue, and green regions, where tissue penetration is much less.

The search for better sensitizers is underway. Much work has centered on efforts to isolate the active component of HPD more precisely (6, 16). However, other classes of compounds may prove superior, and a particularly promising group is the phthalocyanines (4). Many of these have inherent advantages over HPD. They are stable compounds of known structure, relatively easy to synthesize and purify, and often have strong absorption peaks in the appropriate part of the spectrum (600 to 750 nm) with a high yield of singlet oxygen. No major toxic effects have yet been found, and the low absorption at visible wavelengths shorter than 600 nm is likely to reduce the risk of cutaneous photosensitivity, which is a considerable problem with HPD (8, 10). Results so far available suggest that aluminium chlorosulfonated phthalocyanine (AlSPc) has comparable tumor selectivity to HPD and, since this has a strong absorption peak at 675 nm, it appears to be a very promising photosensitizer (31).

The most convenient light sources for PDT are lasers. There are two main reasons for this. Only lasers have a high enough light intensity to get appropriate power levels down small fibers for internal therapy via flexible endoscopes. Secondly, lasers give monochromatic light, so all the energy is delivered at the optimum wavelength for the photosensitizer being used. The most useful lasers are the argon ion pumped dye laser (which is continuous wave) and the copper vapor pumped dye laser (which is a pulsed laser with a high repetition rate, 2 to 20 kc/s). Flash lamp pumped dye lasers, with their low pulse repetition rate, do not seem to be effective (7). It is not yet clear which photosensitizing agent is the best, and since each agent has different absorption peaks, the tunability of the dye laser is a major advantage in the current state of the art. The gold vapor laser has a fixed output at 628 nm, which is ideal for HPD, but because it now seems unlikely that HPD or DHE will be the sensitizer of choice in the future, this is unlikely to the best choice of laser.

Tissue Damage from Photodynamic Therapy

Although PDT has been under careful study in many different centers worldwide for more than 10 years, it is remarkable how little data are available on which factors control the extent of PDT necrosis and what the nature of the tissue damage produced is and how it heals. It is even more remarkable how few studies have been carried out comparing the effects on tumors and on the normal tissue in which those tumors arose. Chaudhuri et al. (11) have shown that PDT can produce extensive sloughing of the jejunal mucosa and submucosa in rats, with sparing of the muscular and serosal layers. Okuda et al. (24) found that extensive necrosis of normal mucosa can occur when treating gastric tumors. In recent work at the National Medical Laser Centre in London, we have tried to elucidate these problems by studying PDT in normal colon and chemically induced colon cancers in rats, following sensitization with AlSPc (3).

These experiments varied the basic parameters involved in PDT (the dose of the photosensitizing drug, the time from photosensitization to light exposure, and the laser power and exposure time). The experimental arrangement was simple. The colon of the rat was exposed at laparotomy and the 0.2 mm fiber delivering the light at 675 nm from an argon ion pumped dye laser was pushed through the wall of the colon into the lumen and held gently against the mucosa of the opposite side. The pharmacodynamics of the sensitizer were assessed by alkali extraction of homogenized specimens of colon taken from animals sensitized at various times before death. The maximum depth of necrosis (seen 2 to 7 days after light exposure) was measured and correlated with the laser parameters, and animals were killed at varying times after treatment for a histologic study of healing. Similar studies were done on rats with colon cancers induced by dimethyl hydrazine (DMH).

The results can be summarized as follows:
- The peak concentration of AlSPc in normal colon occurs 1 hour after administration, whereas the peak in tumors occurs at 48 hours. The maximum ratio, tumor:normal, occurred at 48 hours and was 2.5:1.
- The extent of necrosis for a given light dose varied with the tissue concentration of AlSPc at the time of light exposure. This was true for tumor and normal colon (more detailed quantitative studies have confirmed this in another tumor, a transplantable fibrosarcoma) (32).

– If the laser power is too high (more than 100 mW in these experiments), thermal damage to colon can be just as great as the PDT damage. At 100 mW or less, the depth of PDT damage increases with the applied laser energy on a logarithmic scale.

The biologic effects of thermal and PDT damage were compared (thermal damage being produced with 500 mW laser power in unsensitized animals). The energies were chosen so that full-thickness lesions of comparable width were produced by each technique. Some notable differences were found.

The mechanical strength of treated normal colons was tested by removing the treated section, tying off one end and slowly distending it with gas. As was expected, the strength of thermally damaged bowel was drastically reduced. These sections always burst through the treated area, and the strength only returned to normal after 2 weeks. However, despite extensive full-thickness damage from PDT, there was no reduction whatsoever in the bursting pressure at any time after treatment. Further investigation has shown that this is probably because the collagen in the

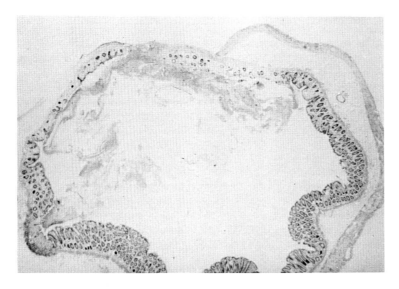

Fig. 1 Thermal damage to normal rat colon 1 day after treatment with a low-power Nd:YAG laser at 1064 nm, showing necrosis of all layers of colon wall
(from K. Matthewson).

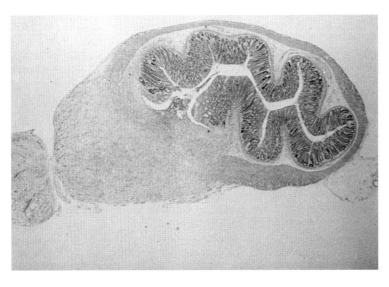

Fig. 2 Similar lesion to Figure 1 showing healing with fibrosis one week after treatment
(from K. Matthewson).

submucosa is damaged by heat but not by PDT (2). On occasion, immediate or delayed spontaneous perforation was seen with the thermal lesions, but this never happened after PDT.

Histologic studies showed that the two types of tissue damage healed differently. Examples of this are shown in Figure 1 to 4. Both excite a marked inflammatory response, but thermal lesions heal with more fibrosis, in contrast to the PDT lesions, which heal with more regeneration of normal tissues. The healing has also been studied in detail in the liver in which it was apparent that the inflammatory response developed much faster after PDT than after thermal damage (12). This is most likely due to the early vascular damage seen

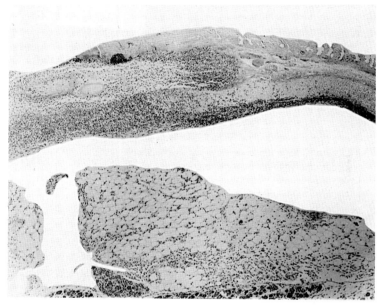

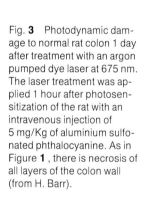

Fig. 3   Photodynamic damage to normal rat colon 1 day after treatment with an argon pumped dye laser at 675 nm. The laser treatment was applied 1 hour after photosensitization of the rat with an intravenous injection of 5 mg/Kg of aluminium sulfonated phthalocyanine. As in Figure 1 , there is necrosis of all layers of the colon wall (from H. Barr).

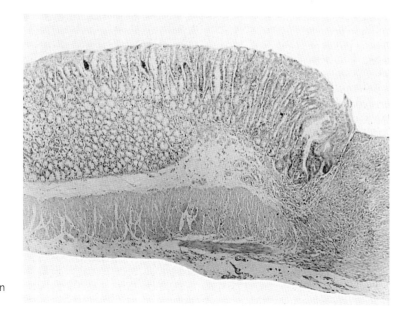

Fig. 4   Similar lesion to Figure 3 , 2 weeks after laser treatment. There is a small area of fibrosis on the right (caused by a local thermal effect where the laser fiber touched the wall of the colon), but the rest of the damaged area has healed with regeneration rather than fibrosis (from H. Barr).

with PDT. Although PDT lesions in normal colon heal by regeneration, tumors necrosed by PDT seem to melt away. However, no detailed studies have yet been carried out to establish what happens at the point where tumors meet normal areas.

A further observation was that colonic bleeding occurred from some of the larger cancers treated by PDT, but not those treated by hyperthermia.

These experimental results can be summarized to give the facts most relevant for clinical use of PDT in the gastrointestinal tract.

1. The extent of necrosis in normal and tumor tissue is predictable and depends on the tissue concentration of photosensitizer at the time of treatment, and the light dose given.
2. There is a maximum ratio of 2.5:1 between the tissue concentration of photosensitizer in tumor and in adjacent normal tissue.
3. Necrosed tumors melt away; necrosed normal bowel heals with regeneration.
4. Hemorrhage may occur after necrosis of larger tumors.

It must also be remembered that no tumor is entirely homogeneous. Solid tumors stimulate an area of neovascularization at their growing front that starts when they are only a few cells' thick (21) and later often develop relatively avascular centers, which may necrose spontaneously. Since PDT seems to have its main effect on vessels, this area of neovascularization should be the prime target, so it is more important to achieve high therapeutic light intensities over the entire growing front of a tumor than its center. Inevitably, this will mean a high light intensity in adjacent normal tissue, with consequent damage to normal areas.

Clinical Applications

As for new treatments in so many branches of medicine and surgery, clinical PDT started on a purely empirical basis with little understanding of the biologic processes involved. The first patients treated were those with multiple cutaneous secondary deposits from tumors such as carcinoma of the breast. Such lesions are readily accessible, easy to monitor after treatment, and serious complications are most

unlikely to develop. However, the published reports of local necrosis in lesions like these are difficult to assess, since there have been no attempts to optimize the tissue concentration of photosensitizer or to adjust the light dose to give necrosis to a depth that matched the extent of the lesions being treated (14).

Empirical treatment of internal tumors is more hazardous. In the early 1980s at the Mayo Clinic a series of ten lung cancers (four superficial, six advanced) were treated by PDT. The four early tumors showed a complete response, but two of those treated for advanced lesions had major intrabronchial hemorrhage 6 and 11 days after PDT, from which they died (13). Such complications have yet to be reported after PDT for gastrointestinal cases, although I am aware of at least two instances, in different countries, in which hemodynamically significant hemorrhage has followed PDT to advanced gastrointestinal tumors. Considering the results of the animal experiments, the most likely explanation for 'this delayed bleeding is that the necrosed tumor sloughs, leaving a raw surface, still in malignant tissue, in which large vessels may be exposed and likely to bleed. However, this can only be fully resolved if the specimens from such cases become available for detailed pathologic study, and no such reports have yet appeared.

These problems should instill caution into any physician contemplating treating advanced tumors with PDT, unless such bleeding can be prevented or easily controlled. McCaughan et al. reported better results with advanced tumors, but they used a mixture of PDT and neodymium:yttrium-aluminum-garnet (Nd: YAG) laser treatments, and the laser power used for PDT was often high enough (1 W) to produce thermal effects in its own right, and so one cannot assess the effect of PDT alone in these cases. The other potential risk of PDT is perforation after necrosis of a tumor which has destroyed all layers of the normal bowel wall, so no collagen is left to maintain the structural integrity of the organ (2).

PDT is far more suitable for early than for advanced tumors. If small tumors necrose and slough after PDT and the resultant defects in the surrounding normal tissue heal by regeneration, there is the potential for eradicating one or many small cancers. Early gastric cancer is far more common in Japan than in Europe, and so it is not surprising that much of the current work on PDT of these lesions comes from Japan. The results are extremely encouraging. In some cases treated by PDT before surgery, no remaining cancer was detectable in the resected specimen (20). However, there are many more problems to overcome before endoscopic PDT can become the treatment of choice for early gastric cancer. The most difficult problem is establishing the true limits of the tumor, both in its lateral extent and its depth of invasion, and knowing whether spread to lymph nodes has occurred. The most promising way of solving this problem is endoscopic ultrasound, which now has good enough resolution to identify each layer of the gastric wall and may also be able to detect enlarged extragastric lymph nodes (9).

When the limits of the cancer have been defined, a technique must be devised to deliver an adequate light dose to every part of the tumor. It is a hopeless task to hold a laser fiber in midair over a gastric lesion and expect to get a predictable light dose at any one point. The fiber will have to be fixed to the tumor in some way so that it does not move during an exposure that may last many minutes. This will be a task for medical physicists to work on in the next few years. Also, the tumor concentration of photosensitizer at the time of phototherapy must be known. This can probably be achieved by chemical extraction techniques on biopsy specimens. It may be sufficiently predictable from the total dose given to the patient and the time from administration to phototherapy, but no data are yet available to test this.

The relative selectivity of PDT together with the lack of scarring on healing might also be of value for treating small multifocal lesions in the colon, such as areas of severe dyplasia or carcinoma in situ in chronic ulcerative colitis or recurrent polyps in the rectum of patients with familial polyposis coli after a colectomy with ileorectal anastomosis. However, these possibilities have not yet been explored.

Conclusion

PDT has considerable promise for the ablation of small single or multifocal tumors in the gastrointestinal tract. Selectivity for malignant areas may not be as great as has been claimed by some PDT enthusiasts, but if normal and malignant areas are necrosed, and both heal by regeneration of normal tissue, then the final result is effectively selective tumor destruction. The technique seems less suitable for advanced cancers, since for these it has no advantage over Nd:YAG laser treatment, and several disadvantages, in particular the need for prior photosensitization (with the possiblity of prolonged cutaneous photosensitivity, especially if the sensitizer used is a porphyrin derivative), and the risk of complications, such as delayed hemorrhage. Nevertheless, the whole field is in a very early stage of development and much research is required to understand the biologic processes involved in PDT and how these can best be used in the treatment of human disease.

References

1. Auler H, Banzer G: Untersuchungen über die Rolle der Porphyrine bei geschwulstkranken Menschen und Tieren. Krebsforschung 53: 65–68, 1942
2. Barr H, Tralau CJ, Boulos PB, MacRobert AJ, Krasner N, Bown SG: Contrasting mechanisms of tissue damage – photodynamic therapy (PDT) preserves collagen, thermal damage does not. Photochem Photobiol 46: 795–800, 1987
3. Barr H, Tralau CJ, MacRobert AJ, Krasner N, Boulos PB, Bown SG: Photodynamic therapy in the normal rat colon with phthalocyanine sensitization. Br J Cancer 56: 111–118, 1987
4. Ben Hur E, Rosenthal: The phthalocyanines: A new class of mammalian cell photosensitizers with a potential for cancer phototherapy. Int J Radiat Biol 47: 145–147, 1985
5. Benson RC: Hematoporphyrin photosensitization and the argon dye laser. In: Smith JA (ed): Lasers in Urologic Surgery. Year Book Medical Publishers, Chicago 1985
6. Berenbaum MC, Bonnett R, Scourides PA: In vivo biological activity of the components of HpD. Br J Cancer 45: 571, 1982
7. Barr H, Boulos PB, MacRobert AJ, Tralau CJ, Phillips D, Bown SG: Comparison of lasers for photodynamic therapy with a phthalocyanine Photosensitiver. Lasers in Med Sci (in press)
8. Bown SG, Tralau CJ, Coleridge Smith PD, Akdemir D, Wieman TJ: Photodynamic therapy with porphyrin and phthalocyanine sensitization: Quantitative studies in normal rat liver. Br J Cancer 54: 43–52, 1986
9. Bugelski PJ, Porter CW, Dougherty TJ: Autoradiographic distribution of HpD in normal and tumor tissue of the mouse. Cancer Res. 41: 4606–4612, 1981
10. Chan WS, Svensen R, Phillips D, Hart IR: Cell uptake, ditribution and response to light of

aluminium sulphonated phthalocyanine, a potential anti-tumour photosensitiser. Br J Cancer 53: 255, 1986

11. Chaudhuri K, Goldblatt PJ, Kreimer-Birnbaum M, Keck RW, Selman SH: Histological study of the effect of HpD photodynamic therapy on the rat jejunum. Cancer Res 46: 2950–2953, 12986

12. Collins CM, Tralau CJ, Wieman TJ, Bown SG: Histological comparison of photodynamic therapy with phthalocyanine sensitisation and thermal injury in normal rat liver. British Medical Laser Association, 4th annual congress, London 1986

13. Cortese DA, Kinsey JH: Endoscopic management of lung cancer with HpD phototherapy. Mayo Clin Proc 57: 543–547, 1982

14. Dahlman A, Wile AG, Burns RG, Mason GR, Johnson FM, Berns MW: Laser photoradiation therapy of cancer. Cancer Res 43: 430–434, 1983

15. Doiron DR, Profio E, Vincent RG, Dougherty TJ: Fluorescence bronchoscopy for detection of lung cancer. Chest 76: 27–32, 1979

16. Dougherty TJ, Potter WR, Weishaupt R: The structure of the active component of HpD. In: Doiron D, Gomer C (eds): Porphyrin Localization and Treatment of Tumors. Alan R Liss, New York 1984 (pp 301–314)

17. Gomer CJ, Dougherty TJ: Determination of ^{3}H and ^{14}C HpD distribution in malignant and normal tissue. Cancer Res 39: 146–151, 1979

18. Gregorie HB, Horger EO, Ward JL, Green JF, Richards T, Robertson HC, Stevenson TB: Hematoporphyrin derivative fluorescence in malignant neoplasms. Ann Surg 167: 820–828, 1968

19. Henderson BW, Waldow SM, Mang TS, Potter WR, Maslone PB, Dougherty TJ: Tumor destruction and kinetics of tumor cell death in two experimental mouse tumors following photodynamic therapy. Cancer Res 45: 572, 1985

20. Kato H, Hawaguchi M, Konaka C: Evaluation of photodynamic therapy in gastric cancer. Lasers Med Sci, 1: 67–74, 1986

21. Kolstad P: The development of the vascular bed in tumours as seen in squamous cell carcinoma of the cervix uteri. Br J Radiol 38: 216–223, 1965

22. Lipson RL, Baldes EJ, Olsen AM: The use of a derivative of hematoporphyrin in tumor detection. J Natl Cancer Inst 26: 1–11, 1961

23. McCaughan JS, Hicks W, Laufman L, May E, Roach R: Palliation of esophageal malignancy with photoradiation therapy. Cancer 54: 2905–2910, 1984

24. Okuda S, Mimura S, Otani T, Ichii M, Tatsuta M: Experimental and clinical studies on HpD photodynamic therapy for upper gastrointestinal cancers. In: Andreoni A, Cubeddu R (eds): Porphyrins in Tumour Phototherapy, 1984 (pp 413–422)

25. Policard A: Etude sur les aspects offerts pour des tumeurs experimentales examines a la lumiere de Wood. C R Soc Biol (Paris) 91: 1423–1424, 1924

26. Selman SH, Kreimer-Birnbaum M, Goldblatt PJ, Anderson TS, Keck RW, Britton SL: Jejunal blood flow after exposure to light in rats injected with HpD. Cancer Res 45: 6425–6427, 1985

27. Spikes JD: Phthalocyanine as photosensitizers in biological systems and for the photodynamic therapy of tumours. Photochem Photobiol 43: 691, 1986

28. Star WM, Marijnissen JPA, van der Berg Blok AE, Reinhold HS: Destructive effect of photoradiation on the microcirculation of a rat mammary tumor growing in 'sandwich' observation channels. In: Doiron D, Gomer C (eds). Porphyrin Localization and Treatment of Tumors. Alan R. Liss, New York 1984 (pp 637–645)

29. Takemoto T, Ito T, Aibe T, Okita K: Endoscopic ultrasonography in the diagnosis of esophageal carcinoma, with particular regard to staging it for operability. Endoscopy 18 (Suppl 3): 22–25, 1986

30. Tappenier H, Jesionek A: Therapeutische Versuche mit fluoreszierenden Stoffen. Muench Med Wochenschr 1: 2042, 1903

31. Tralau CJ, Barr H, Sanderman DR, Barton T, Lewin MR, Bown SG: Aluminium sulphonated phthalocyanine distribution in rodent tumours of the colon, brain and pancreas. Photochem Photobiol 46: 777–781, 1987

32. Tralau CJ, MacRobert AJ, Coleridge-Smith PD, Barr H, Bown SG: Photodynamic therapy with phthalocyanine sensitisation: Quantitative studies in a transplantable fibrosarcoma of rats. Br J Cancer 55: 389–395, 1987

33. Weishaupt KR, Gomer CJ, Dougherty TJ: Identification of singlet oxygen as the cytotoxic agent in photoactivation of a murine tumour. Cancer Res 36: 2326–2329, 1976

34. Wharen RE, Anderson BAS, Laws ER: Quantitation in HpD in human gliomas, experimental central nervous system tumours and normal tissues. Neurosurgery 12: 4446, 1983

Clinical Experiences

R. Lambert, G. Sabben, J. C. Souquet, P. J. Valette, and S. Bonvoisin

Photodynamic therapy, a new method available to oncologists, achieves elective destruction of malignant cells without surgical resection of the tumor. It has been developed progressively from studies on animal models and tissues or cell preparations submitted to irradiation while retaining a photosensitizing agent. Clinical applications in human cancer were stimulated by laser technology, as soon as enough photonic energy could be distributed to the tumor at a specific wavelength.

First clinical applications concerned advanced tumors in patients treated in cancer institutes (cutaneous, inoperable, extension of breast cancer; head and neck inoperable cancer). Elective indications developed shortly after, adapted to certain types of tumors. They concern mainly the lung, the bladder, the cervix, and the upper digestive tract. In each of these specific indications there is a tendency to shift from treatment of advanced to treatment of early cancer. Such cases are usually detected by mass screening or systematic case finding. The method is being developed in centers where there is organized screening. Photodynamic therapy is therefore a stimulant to early detection of cancer; this point has been recently stressed for esophageal cancer (2, 4).

The destruction of cancer cells is based on: injection of a photosensitizing agent in the bloodstream (an hematoporphyrin derivative [HPD]); elective fixation of this agent in the tumor versus the nontumoral tissue after a delay (2 to 3 days); activation of this agent by a specific irradiation (dose, wavelength), followed by an energy transfer to tissue oxygen. The tissue damage results mainly from the cytotoxic effect of the activated "singlet" oxygen on malignant cells and on the vascular system.

Irradiation occurs through a laser source at the specific wavelength 630 nm. This selection results from a compromise between the absorption spectrum of the molecule in the visible light range and the penetration of photons in tissues. Activation of hematoporphyrin requires an energy of 100 to $200 J/cm^2$, with a power density of more than $100 mW/cm^2$. The laser source is either a dye laser circulating the rhodamine B dye and pumped by an argon laser or a pulsed excimer (XeCl) laser (9, 10), or a gold vapor laser directly emitting at 630 nm (25). This amount of energy results in a very moderate temperature increase in the tissue (from 2° to 4°C). This slight elevation potentiates the photobiologic reaction.

Rational of Clinical Application to Digestive Tumors

The efficacy of photodynamic therapy in tumor destruction depends on three main factors:

1. The concentration of the photosensitizing agent in the tumor and its ratio to the concentration in normal tissue. Experimental studies have determined the fixation of HPD in the mucosa and muscularis propria at different levels of the digestive tract (17). The respective concentrations in normal and tumor tissues have been studied as a function of time. Optimal time of irradiation to obtain specific tumor destruction is between 2 and 3 days after injection of the drug. In human observations, the destruction potential of the photobiologic reaction is much higher in squamous cell tumors. This speaks for a higher concentration of HPD in squamous cell tumors than in glandular tumors. It could be explained by the respective cytoplasmic to nuclear ratio in both tissues rather than by differences in vascularization.

2. The depth of invasion of the tumor in the digestive wall, and its relationship to the

penetration of the laser beam in the tissue. Usually complete irradiation of the tumor tissue is possible when the cancer is superficial (limited to mucosa and submucosa). Penetration of the tumor in the muscularis propria introduces high chances of incomplete irradiation of the tumor mass, and, therefore, incomplete destruction. Thus, photodynamic therapy, with a curative objective, is restricted to patients with superficial tumors of the digestive tract.

3. The geometry of irradiation is of utmost importance and a possible cause of failure in the treatment. Small lesions may be adequately or inadequately treated with the same dosimetry, depending on their position and the aiming facility of the laser beam. Irradiation is always easy in the esophagus, whereas a number of "blind" areas occur in the stomach on the lesser curvature or the fundus.

Methods and Results

Patients

From August 1983 to August 1987, we treated 84 patients with photodynamic therapy. The mean age was 70 years. There were 77 men and only 7 women. All patients had tumors of the digestive tract: squamous cell cancer in the esophagus in 51, adenocarcinoma in Barrett's epithelium in the lower esophagus in eight, adenocarcinoma in the cardia obstructing the lower esophagus in seven, adenocarcinoma in the stomach in 16, and adenocarcinoma in the rectum in two. In the early period, patients with advanced cancer were treated; this indication was abandoned due to poor results, and treatment was restricted to patients with tumors classified as superficial at endoscopy. This included 41 patients with squamous cell cancer in the esophagus, three with adenocarcinoma in Barrett's epithelium, and 11 with gastric adenocarcinoma (all other cases had advanced cancer).

Staging of Tumors

Tumors were classified at endoscopy as superficial or advanced. The endoscopic diagnosis of superficial cancer is an assumption based on the following characteristics: absence of stenosis or infiltration; slight alteration in mucosal relief with either a depressed, flat, or elevated pattern. In the esophagus, the flat superficial cancer is detected by staining with the lugol or the toluidine blue method; furthermore, the lesion is often multicentric or multifocal. The endoscopic diagnosis of superficial cancer is supported by other explorations, such as radiography and computed tomography scan; however, validation is possible only after surgical excision and p TNM staging. Staging concerns the depth of invasion in the parietal layers. Mucosal cancers may reach the lamina propria if there is invasion of the muscularis mucosae or if there is a collison and propagation with the ductal epithelium of mucous glands (36). Superficial cancers are limited to the mucosa and submucosa. In the absence of lymphatic invasion a superficial cancer is classified as early. Actually, there is no validation of the classification in nonoperated patients; this includes most of the patients treated by photodynamic therapy and classified as superficial at endoscopy.

The best approach to preoperative staging of the tumor is endoscopic ultrasonography (EUS). Since March 1986, we examined all patients with an endoscopic diagnosis of superficial cancer with the Olympus EUUM2 echoendoscope (transducer emitting at 7.5 MHz) with a water-filled balloon surrounding the tip of the endoscope in the esophagus. The echoic pattern of the esophageal wall allowed identification of the second hyperechoic layer with the submucosa and of the second hypoechoic layer with the muscularis propria. Therefore, the critical distinction between superficial and nonsuperficial cancer was possible at this level. The tumor was identified through its hypoechoic pattern interfering with the hyperechoic layers. Lymph nodes in the mediastinum were classified, according to shape, size, and echoic pattern, as normal or malignant. In the stomach the exploration was based on similar criteria. Efficacy in staging versus treatment selection was tested in 25 patients and was confirmed in 24. Efficacy in assessment of tumor recurrence or persistence in the esophagus was tested in 26 explorations conducted in 20 patients, and concordance between EUS and endoscopy findings was good in 21.

Treatment Selection

All patients with *advanced cancer* in the esophagus, stomach, or rectum were inoperable due to inextirpability of the tumor, old age, or associated diseases.

In patients with an *endoscopic pattern of superficial cancer* the decision analysis was more complex.

1. The choice between the surgical or nonsurgical approach was based on the physical condition of the patient, age, acceptance of or opposition to operation.
2. When a nonsurgical protocol was adopted in squamous cell cancer of the esophagus, the following elements of treatment were listed: thermal photodestruction by neodymium:yttrium-aluminum-garnet (Nd:YAG) laser (5, 6), photobiologic nonthermal destruction after injection of hematoporphyrin (18, 19, 20) chemotherapy (21) with sessions, such as cisplatin $100 \, mg/m^2$ for one day, 5-fluororouracil (5-FU) $1 \, g/m^2$ for four days. Radiotherapy (21) at a 60 Gy dose, administered in 2 or 3 sessions.

The patients were managed as follows: *superficial cancer confirmed* (muscularis propria unaltered), photodynamic therapy; *superficial cancer unconfirmed* (invasion of the muscularis at EUS), Nd:YAG laser thermal destruction. A combined protocol with laser plus chemotherapy and radiotherapy was proposed in both groups of patients when their physical condition was good and their age less than 70 years.

In the photodynamic therapy protocol, the sequence was as follows: laser photodestruction with 2 months delay to avoid additive toxic effects of combined treatments, then radiotherapy with or without chemotherapy. In the Nd:YAG protocol the sequence was as follows: initial chemotherapy session, photodestruction of the endoluminal tumor, and then radiotherapy.

3. When a nonsurgical protocol was adopted in a patient with a gastric adenocarcinoma classified as superficial at endoscopy, the respective indications of photodynamic therapy and Nd:YAG laser were the same as for the esophagus; however, combined protocol with chemotherapy and radiotherapy was not administered.
4. For both types of tumor, an accurate protocol selection was possible through EUS staging since March 1986. Before this period, the selection of cases for photody-

namic therapy was based only on the endoscopic pattern.

Photodynamic Therapy: the Methodology

The *photosensitizing agent* was administered intravenously within a pressure infusion. In the first cases it was an HPD (from Oncology Research and Development), Photofrin I, injected with a dose of 3.0 to 3.5 mg/kg. Later, we used the dihematoporphyrin ether (DHE) (Photomedica Co.) with a dose of 2.0 to 2.5 mg/kg. The drug was kept frozen until the preparation for injection.

Irradiation of the tumor in the digestive tract occurred after a delay of 2 to 3 days. Most patients had only a single session of irradiation after injection of the drug. However, when the tumor destruction was estimated to be incomplete (at 24 hours), a second irradiation was done. The time between injection and the second irradiation never exceeded 6 days. The source of the 630 nm laser beam was a SP dye laser circulating rhodamine B and pumped by an argon SP laser. The power obtained varied from 700 to 1000 mW at the tip of the flexible quartz fiber transmitting the laser beam. This fiber was introduced into the operative channel of a fiberscope. An optical dispatcher was positioned at the end of the tip, ensuring a lateral emission of the beam as a narrow 180° or 360°C rim, according to the model. Therefore, the power density during irradiation of the tumor reached around $300 \, mW/cm^2$. The amount of energy density distributed to the tumor varied from 100 to $200 \, J/cm^2$. The time of irradiation varied according to the surface of the tumor, from 5 to 30 min.

Follow-up

During 1 month after the session, the patients were asked to avoid any direct exposure to sunlight. However, they could return home within 2 days after the treatment, and some of them were treated as outpatients. On average, the prevention of cutaneous intolerance was effective, well accepted, and compatible with a normal life for retired persons. The endoscopic follow-up of the lesion was undertaken 24 hours after irradiation, at 2 weeks and 1 month in the early period. When malignant tissue persisted at the end of 1 month (incomplete response), the result was classified as failure. In some patients the surgical alternative was reconsidered; others underwent a second episode of photodynamic therapy with injection of a new dose of drug. Later, the follow-up was conducted at 3-months intervals.

Combined protocols were adopted for 50% of patients with squamous cell cancer in the esophagus, when their physical condition was compatible with chemotherapy sessions (cisplatin and 5-FU) and radiotherapy. An interval of 2 months was maintained between the injection of photofrin and the first session of radiotherapy.

Photodynamic Therapy: Efficacy and Tolerance

Tumor destruction began a few hours after irradiation with the following steps: swelling and congestion of the tissue with vasodilation during the first 24 hours; necrosis beginning at 48 hours; elimination of necrotic tissue; tissue repair with or without tumor regrowth. The length of evolution was reduced to a few days in superficial epithelial cancer, whereas necrosis persisted from 1 to 3 months in advanced cancer.

During the first 24 hours, *mild chest pain* was observed in 50% of patients receiving treatment in the esophagus. It was associated with tissue inflammation.

Tolerance was on average excellent. Transient and mild cutaneous reactions of photosensitiziation were observed in seven patients who did not respect the contraindication to sun exposure. Furthermore, among patients treated with a combined protocol, severe radiodermatitis was observed in four patients who had been submitted to radiotherapy only 4 weeks after the injection of the photosensitizing agent. Prolonging the delay resulted in complete prevention of this side-effect. In two other patients on a combined protocol a reversible bone marrow aplasia was observed, related to chemotherapy.

Results in Squamous Cell Cancer in the Esophagus

In the first 10 patients with *advanced cancer* treated by this method a response was observed in all, but with incomplete tumor destruction; regrowth occurred after 1 to 2

months. Furthermore, the symptomatic effect was poor due to chronic elimination of necrosis in the esophageal lumen, resulting in obstruction. Results in palliation were not as good as with Nd:YAG photodestruction.

Therefore, indications were restricted to *superficial cancer* as detected at endoscopy (and confirmed at EUS for the last cases). The 41 treated patients included 37 men and four women. Associated cancers were present in 11 (of which five were in the mouth, pharynx, and bronchial tree). Of the 41 patients, 27 were new and untreated cases, and 14 had recurrent tumors after previous treatment. Follow-up was conducted in 39 patients (20 in monotherapy, 19 in a combined protocol; the two other cases have just been treated. The efficacy of tumor destruction was estimated in 37 patients with biopsies of the tumor site. Negative biopsies were obtained in 32 patients (86%) and in five patients incomplete destruction was affirmed (1 to 5 months after treatment). Of the 32 lesions with complete destruction, biopsies remained negative during the follow-up (2 to 40 months) in 28. In four a recurrence was observed (at 9, 11, 22, and 24 months) and was treated by photodynamic therapy. Of the 39 patients included in the follow-up, 27 are alive (average, 14.8 months) and 12 are dead (average, 9.6 months). Death was related to cancer evolution in four, and unrelated in 8. The actuarial survival rate taking into account all cases of mortality was 50% at 16 months. The probability of surviving patients remaining disease-free is 65% at 16 months and 52% at 24 months.

Results in Esophageal Adenocarcinoma in Barrett's Epithelium

In five patients with tumors at an *advanced stage,* prompt recurrence after incomplete destruction was observed; furthermore, inflammation and fibrosis resulted in a narrow stenosis, difficult to manage. In three patients with cancer classified as superficial at endoscopy, incomplete destruction was also obtained. In one patient the follow-up reached 24 months and the treatment shifted to palliation by repeated Nd:YAG laser sessions; in the other patient complete destruction was obtained with recurrence 5 months later; in the third patient exeresis was performed after a 5-month interval.

Results in Gastric Adenocarcinoma

In 12 patients with *advanced cancer* (seven located at the cardia, five in the stomach) an incomplete response with prompt tumor regrowth was obtained. The symptomatic benefit was considered as nil. In 11 patients with a gastric cancer considered to be superficial at endoscopy, complete response with negative biopsies at the site of the lesion was obtained. However, recurrence occurred after a delay of 12 to 18 months, requiring further treatment (repeated photodynamic therapy or Nd:YAG laser sessions). Most of these patients were asymptomatic, tolerance of the treatment was good, and the longest follow-up reached 4 years.

Results in Colorectal Adenocarcinoma

In two patients with an advanced nonoperable cancer of the rectum, a partial response was obtained with no influence on symptoms and evolution.

Indications

Squamous Cell Cancer in the Esophagus

In the literature, in addition to our own data, results of treatment of advanced squamous cell cancer in the esophagus have been published as very small (usually less than 10 cases) series in Japan (16, 27), China (11, 22, 35), Australia (37), Europe (32, 38), and the United States (23, 24). Incomplete destruction of the tumor was always the result: therefore, preference should be given in palliation to laser destruction with the Nd:YAG laser, as the simplest and most efficient procedure.

As for squamous cell cancer at the superficial stage, acceptable results have been obtained in Japan (28, 30, 34), Europe (ourselves) and the United States (7, 8). As an example three cases out of six treated by Okushima et al. (30) are alive and disease-free at 2 years; five cases of seven treated by Okitsu et al. (28) are disease-free after 20 to 57 months. The power of the laser beam during irradiation should be adapted to the depth of invasion of the tumor in order to increase the percentage of complete responses (31).

1. Photodynamic therapy can be recommended as an elective treatment of superficial esophageal cancer when there is a good demonstration of the integrity of the muscularis propria (EUS staging). The protocol is in monotherapy if the patient is old or in poor health. It must be completed by radiotherapy and possibly chemotherapy if the patient is less than 70 years old and in good health.
2. When there is doubt about the classification (no EUS staging, uncertain EUS interpretation), there is a choice between the two protocols based on Nd:YAG laser or photodynamic therapy.
3. If there is no doubt about a large muscular invasion by the tumor, photodynamic therapy is contraindicated.

Adenocarcinoma in the Esophagus

This includes adenocarcinoma of the cardia obstructing the lower esophagus or adenocarcinoma developed in a Barrett's epithelium. Very few cases have been reported in the literature (22–24, 33, 37) and often not separated from squamous cell cancers. Results were poor and responses incomplete as in our series. This method is contraindicated in advanced cancer. Furthermore, in all three cases of superficial cancer in Barrett's epithelium from our series we obtained an incomplete response.

Adenocarcinoma in the Stomach

Data have been published about application of the method to advanced cancer (14, 24), Results are poor, and treatment should focus on superficial gastric cancer as detected at endoscopy. Most data have been published in Japan (13–15, 26, 29, 34). The rate of complete responses at endoscopy is very high: 10 of 13 for Kato et al. (14), 70% for Okuda and Mimura (29). The depth of invasion of the tumor plays a role; the rate of complete responses is estimated at 67% for intramucosal lesions and 28% for lesions extending to the submucosa (13). However, the rate of complete responses is much lower when the tumor destruction is controlled in the operative specimen: six cases of 13 for Kato et al. (14). Ogura and Tajiri (26) reported in 1986 global results of the Japanese experience: 89 cases of early gastric cancer were treated with pending results on 55, complete destruction with negative biopsies at 1 year in 29, and confirmed recurrence before 1 year in 5. In summary, photodynamic therapy is an elegant and elective treatment of superficial gastric cancer, but the rate of complete tumor destruction is not high enough to justify the method in operable patients.

Adenocarcinoma in the Colon and Rectum

A few experimental data concern the tissue concentration of the HPD in normal and neoplastic colonic tissue in humans as well as its fluorescence (1, 39). Therapeutic application (12, 16, 27, 32) does not seem to deserve further developments. Indeed, superficial cases are adequately treated by resection or Nd:YAG laser photodestruction, whereas poor results are expected from palliation in advanced cases.

References

1. Bottiroli G, Dal Fante M, Spinelli S: Comparative analysis of HPD fluorescence in adenoma and adenocarcinoma of the bowel. Third Congress of ELA. Amsterdam, November 6–8, 1986 (p 74)
2. Dancygier H, Classen M: How can we diagnose the depth of cancer invasion in the esophagus? Endoscopy 18: 19–21, 1986
3. Dougherty TJ: Photodynamic therapy. In: Jori G, Perria C (eds): Photodynamic Therapy of Tumors and Other Diseases. Padova 1985, Edizioni Libreria Progetto (pp 267–280)
4. Endo M, Takeshita K, Yoshida M: How can we diagnose the early stage of esophageal cancer? Endoscopic diagnosis. Endoscopy 18: 11–18, 1986
5. Fleischer D: Endoscopic palliative tumour therapy with laser irradiation. Clin Gastroenterol 15: 273–278, 1986
6. Fleischer D, Sivak MV: Endoscopic Nd YAG laser therapy as palliation for esophagogastric cancer. Parameters affecting initial outcome. Gastroenterology 89: 827–831, 1985
7. Gluckman JL: The role of photodynamic therapy in the management of early cancers of the upper aerodigestive tract. First International Conference on the Clinical Applications of Photosensitization for Diagnosis and Treatment, Tokyo, April 30 – May 2, 1986 (p 71)
8. Gluckman JL, Weissler MC: Role of photodynamic therapy in the management of early cancers of the upper aerodigestive tract. Lasers Med Sci 1: 217–220, 1986
9. Hirano T, Ishida K, Yasukawa M et al: Cancer diagnosis system using HPD and excimer-dye laser. In Jori G, Perria C (eds): Photodynamic Therapy of Tumors and Other Diseases. Edizioni Libreria Progetto, 1985 (pp. 325–328)
10. Hirano T, Ishizuka M, Watuka T, et al: Cancer treatment with an excimer dye laser. First International Conference on the Clinical Applications of Photosensitization for Diagnosis and Treatment, Tokyo, April 30 – May 2, 1986 (p 91)
11. Jin M: Analysis of hematoporphyrin derivative (HPD) and laser photodynamic therapy of upper gastrointestinal tumors in 52 cases. First International Conference on the Clinical Applications of Photosensitization for Diagnosis and Treatment, Tokyo, April 30 – May 2, 1986 (p 72)
12. Kamaya A, Ito Y, Kano T, et al: Endoscopic photodynamic therapy of colorectal adenoma and carcinoma. First International Conference on the Clinical Applications of Photosensitization for Diagnosis and Treatment, Tokyo, April 30 – May 2, 1986 (p 156)
13. Kasugai T, Ito Y, Kameya A, et al: Endoscopic photodynamic therapy of early gastric cancer. First International Conference on the Clinical Applications of Photosensitization for Diagnosis and Treatment. Tokyo, April 30 – May 2, 1986 (p 48)
14. Kato H, Kawaguchi M, Konaka C, et al: Evaluation of photodynamic therapy in gastric cancer. Lasers Med Sci 1: 67–74, 1986
15. Kinoshita K, Kawate N, Sakai H, et al: PDT in early gastric cancer. Frist International Conference on the Clinical Applications of Photosensitization for Diagnosis and Treatment, Tokyo, April 30 – May 2, 1986 (p 141)
16. Kouzu T, Konno H, Isono K: Estimation and future development of photodynamic therapy for digestive tract cancer. First International Conference on the Clinical Applications of Photosensitization for Diagnosis and Treatment, Tokyo, April 30 – May 2, 1986 (p 139)
17. Kusumoto K, Wada K, Konno K, et al: Change of HPD distribution in digestive organs. First International Conference on the Clinical Applications of Photosensitization for Diagnosis and Treatment, Tokyo, April 30 – May 2, 1986 (p 126)
18. Lambert R, Sabben G: Cancer in the esophagus: Treatment by photoradiation therapy. Lasers Surg Med 3: 341, 1984
19. Lambert R, Sabben G, Souquet JC, et al: Esophageal squamous cell cancer: Indications for photodynamic therapy. First International Conference on the Clinical Applications of Photosensitization for Diagnosis and Treatment, Tokyo, April 30 – May 2, 1986 (p 73)
20. Lambert R, Sabben G, Souquet JC, et al: Photodynamic therapy in superficial squamous cell cancer of the esophagus. Third Congress of ELA, Amsterdam, November 6–8 1986 (p 114)
21. Leichman L, Herskovic A, Leichman CG et al: Nonoperative therapy for squamous-cell cancer of the esophagus. J Clin Oncol 5: 365–370, 1987
22. Li J, Guan D, Zhao S, Wang F, et al: Photodynamic therapy in upper gastrointestinal malignant tumors. First International Conference on the Clinical Applications of Photosensitization for Diagnosis and Treatment, Tokyo, April 30 – May 2, 1986 (p 140)

23. McCaughan JS: Observations from the treatment of 182 patients with photodynamic therapy. First International Conference on the Clinical Applications of Photosensitization for Diagnosis and Treatment, Tokyo, April 30 – May 2, 1986 (p 157)

24. McCaughan JS, Hicks W, Laufman L, et al: Palliation of esophageal malignancy with photoradiation therapy. Cancer 54: 2905–2910, 1984

25. McKenzie AL, Carruth JAS: A comparison of gold-vapour and dye lasers for photodynamic therapy. Lasers Med Sci 1: 117–120, 1986

26. Oguro Y, Tajiri H: Endoscopic laser treatment of G. I. tract cancer in Japan. Update. Communication at the 8th World Congress of Gastroenterology, Sao Paulo 1986

27. Ohuchi T, Kato K, Nakajima A, et al: PDT in recurrent rectal carcinoma using a pulsed gold vapor laser. First International Conference on the Clinical Applications of Photosensitization for Diagnosis and Treatment, Tokyo, April 30 – May 2, 1986 (p 78)

28. Okitsu H, Hayata Y, Kato H, et al: Photodynamic therapy with hematoporphyrin derivative in esophageal cancer. First International Conference on the Clinical Applications of Photosensitization for Diagnosis and Treatment, Tokyo, April 30 – May 2, 1986 (p 75)

29. Okuda S, Mimura S: HPD photodynamic therapy for early gastric cancer. First International Conference on the Clinical Applications of Photosensitization for Diagnosis and Treatment, Tokyo, April 30 – May 2, 1986 (p 47)

30. Okushima N, Ide H, Hanyu F, et al: Photodynamic therapy in early stage cancer of the esophagus. First International Conference on the Clinical Applications of Photosensitization for Diagnosis and Treatment, Tokyo, April 30 – May 2, 1986 (p 46)

31. Okushima N, Yoshida M, Fukui H, et al: Photodynamic therapy of esophageal cancer with particular attention to histopathological aspects. First International Conference on the Clinical Applications of Photosensitization for Diagnosis and Treatment, Tokyo, April 30 – May 2, 1986 (p 102)

32. Patrice T, Jutel P, Foultier MT, et al: Photochemotherapy mediated by hematoporphyrin derivative in gastroenterology. Eur J Cancer Clin Oncol 23: 509–512, 1987

33. Sabben G, Maiza E, Lambert R, et al: PDT in adenocarcinoma of the upper digestive tract. First International Conference on the Clinical Applications of Photosensitization for Diagnosis and Treatment, Tokyo, April 30 – May 2, 1986 (p 136)

34. Shiotani H, Tajiri H, Oguro Y, et al: Current report of photodynamic therapy for cancer of the esophagus and stomach. First International Conference on the Clinical Applications of Photosensitization for Diagnosis and Treatment, Tokyo, April 30 – May 2, 1986 (p 74)

35. Song SZ, Li JH, Zou J, et al: Hematoporphyrin derivative and laser photodynamical reaction in the diagnosis and treatment of malignant tumors. Lasers Surg Med 5: 61–66, 1985

36. Takubo K, Takai A, Takayama S, et al: Intraductal spread of eosphageal squamous cell carcinoma. Cancer 59: 1751–1757, 1987

37. Thomas RJS, Morstyn G, St John DJB, et al: Photoradiation treatment of esophageal cancer. First International Conference on the Clinical Applications of Photosensitization for Diagnosis and Treatment, Tokyo, April 30 – May 2, 1986 (p 45)

38. Tomio L, Corti L, Norberto L, et al: Photodynamic therapy with hematoporphyrin in cancer of esophagus. Third Congress of ELA, Amsterdam, November 6–8, 1986 (p 76)

39. Wooten RS, Ahlquist DA, Carpenter HA, et al: Localization of hematoporphyrin derivative in colorectal neoplasia. Lasers Surg. Med 6: 192, 1986

State of the Art in Photodynamic Therapy

P. Spinelli

The ideal therapy for tumors is one that removes malignant tissue without damage ot the host. Photodynamic therapy (PDT) is an experimental therapy for solid tumors based on selectivity, the ideal principle of cancer treatment.

The principle of selectivity is inspiring the new techniques and continuously improving results of surgery, with more and more conservative operations, radiotherapy, more interest in methods of precise and localized irradiation and in afterloading techniques, and with chemotherapy, selecting drugs with marked tumor affinity. PDT, based on the interaction of a photosensitizer and of an activating light in the presence of oxygen, has the necessary premises to satisfy requirements of selectivity, and, in some accurately selected patients, of radicality.

Fields of application for PDT: *Skin:* Indication for PDT is extensive; multicentric or critically sited primary cancers, in patients for whom traditional methods of treatment are considered inappropriate (2). Also cutaneous and subcutaneous metastases from breast carcinoma have been treated.

Gynecological tumors (10): Primary vaginal carcinoma, especially when located in the upper third, is difficult to treat with conventional methods because the anatomic relationship to the rectum and bladder can cause fistulas. Superficially infiltrating carcinomatous ulcers of the vulva, regardless of diameter have been treated. Intraepithelial cancer of the uterine cervix has been treated. The problem of the possible involvement of the deep parts of the cervical glands in the neoplastic process remains, and the effectiveness of PDT in completely destroying the cervical glands must yet be demonstrated.

Head and neck: Cutaneous and mucosal cancers in this area, especially when found in critical positions, have been treated. Cases of face, tongue, nasopharynx, larynx, and vocal cord carcinomas have been reported as responding to PDT (1).

Eye: Various interesting applications for PDT have been proposed in ophthalmologic treatment. Malignant melanoma of the choroid and retinoblastoma responded to therapy. In the case of highly pigmented melanomas a thermal effect is suspected to be a very important therapeutic factor owing to the high quantity of energy used to treat these lesions. Particular indications, such as control of lens epithelial proliferation secondary to cataract surgery, have been recently proposed (8).

Brain (6): Clinical studies involving patients with malignant brain tumors irradiated on the surface or by fiber optic implantation both stereotactically or surgically have been reported, but it is too early to assess the results. Photosensitizers can be administered topically or intravenously.

Vascular system: Atheromatous plaques show porphyrin uptake (4). It can be demonstrated by fluorescence methods (violet light illumination). This is probably due to the rich vascularization of human plaques that allows porphyrin to reach the plaques, but also other, different mechanisms may be involved in the absorption of the photosensitizer by atheromatous plaques. The clinical importance of this could lead to using PDT in arteries occluded by atheromas, by removing or reducing plaques, using methods of treatment similar to those used for PDT in other areas of the body. However, even if PDT appears efficacious for atheromas, many problems will arise in the clinical applications.

Endoscopic treatment: PDT has demonstrated particular usefulness in endoscopic treatments (12), especially in cases of small tumors with macroscopically undefined borders or in cases of multicentric tumors. These conditions are mostly present in the upper and lower digestive tract, in the bronchi, and in the bladder. Hayata et al. at Tokyo Medical College started with clinical endoscopic applications of PDT in 1980 and have now accumulated the largest experience in the world in the various fields.

International Inquiries

In two international inquiries proposed in 1984 and in 1986, we collected data from 467 and 912 patients, respectively (Figs. **1–4**). The inquiries suggest that the number of centers working with PDT is increasing. Geographically, the centers expanded all over the world during the last years. Up to 1984, 467 patients had been treated in eight centers, between 1984 and 1986 the total number increased to 912 and the number of centers to 20. The laser sources used show that four groups are using the new gold vapor lasers and that activation by neodymium:yttrium-aluminum-garnet (Nd:YAG) laser photoradiation has been

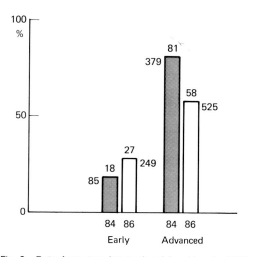

Fig. 1 Data from two international inquiries in 1984 and 1986 on laser types.

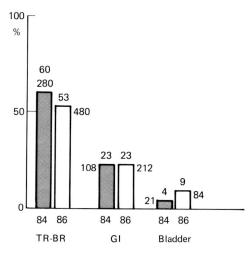

Fig. 2 Data from two international inquiries in 1984 and 1986 on anatomic site of treated lesions. TR-BR : tracheobronchial; GI: gastrointestinal.

Fig. 3 Data from two international inquiries in 1984 and 1986 on stage of the tumor.

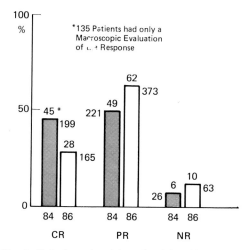

Fig. 4 Data from two international inquiries in 1984 and 1986 on response of patients to laser therapy.

abandoned. Practically unchanged are the photosensitizers used, the time interval between drug injection and irradiation, and the modality of irradiation. Regarding the anatomic areas irradiated, the number of bladder treatments is increasing. Regarding the stage, early tumors are preferred to advanced ones. The power and the energy of treatments tend to increase, probably because of a relative optimization of treatment parameters. If the overall results are considered, they may appear worse in the last than in the previous inquiry, but we must take into account that 135 patients from the previous inquiry were referred to as complete response (CR) after only a macroscopic evaluation (for example: the reopening of a bronchus). The results of the last (1986) inquiry show a CR in 61% of early stage and in 7% of advanced tumors treated, partial response (PR) in 33% early and 80% advance, and no response (NR) in 6% early and 13% advanced.

Perspectives

After a very promising beginning, showing responsiveness to PDT by most human solid tumors, we now expect a relative restraint in clinical application and more activity in basic research.

Actually, many reasons make a reevaluation of PDT necessary; regarding the perspectives of PDT one must sort out the most important problems: photosensitizers, laser light, and therapeutic combination protocols.

Photosensitizers

The most common photosensitizers are hematoporphyrin derivative (HPD) and dihematoporphyrin ether or ester (DHE), its active form. These drugs have two limitations: skin photosensitization and low tissue penetration of the light at the wavelength used for the activation of the sensitizer (11). Skin photosensitization presents a real limitation to the possibilities of treatment especially into outpatients clinics because the drug may remain in the body for 3 to 4 weeks after injection. The solution may be found in local administration of the photosensitizer (9), which is very difficult for noncutaneous lesions, or in finding a more selective drug and consequently using smaller amounts, reducing cutaneous sensitization. Furthermore, new drugs, now in the

experimental stage, with a high absorption coefficient in the near infrared would improve light penetration into the tumor (5). Among the new drugs, some are compounds resulting from modification of porphyrins: modifying the structure of DHE by converting one or more of the porphyrin rings to chlorin (DHEC), and linking hematoporphyrin to chlorin. Of great interest is also the use of phthalocyanines, which are porphyrin-like compounds with a main absorption band in the red. Experiments have shown them to be very efficient as photosensitizers. The effective spectrum for chloraluminium phthalocyanine (CAPC) is a narrow band centered around 680 nm, CAPC appears to be about 50 times more efficient than HPD and the shift of its action spectrum to the red allows for better light penetration into the irradiated tumors. The doses of this drug can be much lower than HPD and DHE and from 0.2 to 0.5 mg/kg of body weight, because phthalocyanines absorb a larger number of photons. They tend to from aggregates and are bound to lipoproteins; 24 hours after injection the maximum host-tumor gradient can be found. Phthalocyanines are eliminated with the bile without metabolic modifications. Unlike porphyrins, phthalocyanines would induce limited damage to the vascular endothelium, so maintaining the blood-oxygen supply to the tumor during the treatment.

New Lasers and Irradiation Modalities

New laser devices are actually under study; of special interest are tunable dye lasers, which can produce different wavelengths, and new modalities of irradiation by short pulses.

Selection of Patients and Combined Protocols

Indications for PDT are changing since the first attempts. PDT seems to be more reliable in treating small cancer lesions, superficially extended on large areas, and multicentric. PDT can be used for curative and for palliative treatment. It can treat cancer at various stages, from precancerous lesions to cancer in situ and invasive cancer both at early (13) and at advanced stages (7). The future tendency is to develop treatment in the field of early cancer and precancerous lesions. Treatment protocols, involving combination of traditional therapies, are now being submitted for international evaluation.

References

1. Carruth JAS, McKenzie AL: Pilot study of photo-dynamic therapy for the treatment of superficial tumors of the skin and head and neck. In: Jori G, Perria C (eds): Photodynamic Therapy of Tumors and Other Diseases. Progetto Publ, Padova 1985 (p 289)
2. Gregory RO, Goldman L: Application of PDT in plastic surgery. Lasers Surg Med 6: 62, 1986
3. Hayata Y, Kato H, Konaka C, Ono J, Takizawa N: Hematoporphyrin derivative and laser photoradiation in the treatment of lung cancer. Chest 81: 269, 1981
4. Kessel D, Sykes E: Porphyrin accumulation by atheromatous plaques of the aorta. Photochem Photobiol 40: 59, 1984
5. Kol R, Ben-Hur E, Riklis E, Marko R, Rosenthal I: Photosensitized inhibition of mitogenic stimulation of human lymphocytes by aluminium phthalocyanine tetrasulphonate. Laser Med Sci 1: 187, 1986
6. Laws ER, Wharen RE, Anderson RE: Photodynamic therapy of brain tumors. In Jori G, Perria C (eds): Photodynamic Therapy of Tumors and other Diseases. Progetto Publ. Padova 1985 (p 311)
7. McCaughan JS, Williams TE, Bethel BH: Palliation of esophageal malignancy with photodynamic therapy. Ann Thor Surg 40: 113, 1985
8. Parel JM, Cubeddu R, Ramponi R, Lingua R, Sacchi CA, Haefliger E: Endocapsular rinsing with Photofrin II as a photodynamic therapy for lens epithelial proliferation. (Abstr.) Third Congress of ELA. Lasers Med, Sci 1: 289, 1986
9. Sacchini V, Melloni E, Marchesini R, Luini A, Bandieramonte G, Spinelli P, Cascinelli N: Preliminary clinical studies with PDT by topical TPPS administration in neoplastic skin lesions. Laser Surg Med 7: 6, 1987
10. Soma H, Nutahara S: Cancer of the female genitalia in lasers and hematoporphyrin derivative. In Hayata Y,. Dougherty TJ (eds): Lasers and Hematoporphyrin Derivative in Cancer. Igaku-Shoin, Tokyo 1983 (p 97)
11. Spikes JD, Jori G: Photodynamic therapy of tumours and other diseases using porphyrins. Laser Med Sci 2: 3, 1987
12. Spinelli P: Endoscopic laser-fluorescence and photochemotherapy of cancer. Acta Endosc 13: 201, 1983
13. Tajiri H, Daizukono N, Joffe SN, Oguro Y: Photoradiation therapy in early gastrointestinal cancer. Gastrointest Endosc 33: 88, 1987

Combined Therapy with Laser

Laser and Afterloading Radiation with Iridium-192

F. Hagenmüller, C. Sander, R. Sander, G. Ries, and M. Classen

The most widespread methods for the endoscopic palliation of malignant obstruction of the esophagus and the cardia are radiation with laser light and insertion of endoprostheses. The most important advantage of endoscopic laser therapy is its high efficacy and safety (2). However, the value of laser treatment is limited by the necessity for repeated endoscopic procedures at 3- to 4-week intervals. This leaves the patient dependent on the endoscopist and impairs his quality of life. The endoscopic implantation of an esophageal endoprosthesis can mostly be performed as a one-step procedure necessitating only a few days hospitalization of the patient. The endoprosthesis can overcome not only the luminal obstruction, but also cover an esophagobronchial fistula. A disadvantage of prosthesis insertion is the remarkable rate of acute (5 to 30%) and long-term (7 to 34%) complications (3). The procedure-related mortality of esophageal endoprosthesis implantation ranges up to 12.8% (3).

To overcome these limitations of endoscopic laser therapy and prosthesis placement for the palliation of inoperable carcinomas of the esophagus and cardia, the combination of laser therapy with endoluminal radiation with iridium-192 was introduced (1). This concept was introduced to take advantage of the low complication rate of laser therapy and to prolong the palliative effect when compared with laser therapy alone.

Method

The method is applied in patients with obstruction of the esophagus and the cardia due to inoperable carcinomas.

The initial therapeutic step is laser radiation of the tumor obstruction. It is performed with a continuous wave neodymium:yttrium-aluminum-garnet (Nd:YAG) laser (Medilas, MBB- Medizintechnik GmbH, Munich) with a wavelength of 1.06 µm and an output power of 100 W. Laser therapy is performed at 2-day intervals until the tumor stenosis can be passed with an endoscope. Thereafter, endoluminal radiation with iridium-192 is carried out. The radioactive iridium is guided into the tumor stenosis through an application tube. This tube has an outer diameter of 4 mm and is made of Teflon. Its distal tip must be placed, under endoscopic control, at the lower end of the tumor stenosis of the esophagus or the cardia. The application tube is led out through the nose and fixed. After placement of the application tube, the patient enters a radiation-protected room where the radioactive source is kept in a metal-shielded container (Gammamed II, Sauerwein Company, West Germany). The external end of the application tube is attached to the source container. The physician may now leave the radiation-protected room. The patient can be observed from outside by means of a video camera. The iridium-192 wire is advanced into the distal end of the application tube by remote control (afterloading technique). It stays in place until the dose of 7 Gy has been applied at a depth of 1 cm from the radiation source. Then the iridium wire is withdrawn in 1 cm decrements within the tumor stenosis until the whole length of the stenosis has been radiated. The duration of radiation at each station within the tumor can be precalculated according to the activity of the radiation source. Usually, the radiation exposure does not take longer than 30 minutes. When the whole tumor stenosis has been irradiated, the iridium wire and the application tube are removed.

Depending on the effect, the radiation can be repeated up to five times. The first three applications are performed at 1-week-intervals. Further irradiation is carried out only in case of recurrent stenosis due to tumor growth during the follow-up.

Endoluminal iridium radiation can be performed on an outpatient basis.

Patient Selection

The combined therapy with laser and endoluminal iridium-192 radiation can be applied in patients with inoperable malignant obstructions of the esophagus and the cardia. It is an alternative to bougienage, prosthesis implantation, and laser therapy alone. The assessment of inoperability should always be a matter of interdisciplinary discussion between the internist and an experienced surgeon.

Esophagobronchial fistula is a contraindication for combined laser and iridium radiation. Patients with esophageal carcinomas less than 2 cm in length without detectable metastases and inoperability due to their general condition should receive external radiation because these candidates have a small chance of cure. In such cases, endoluminal iridium radiation can be added in order to boost the effect of the external radiation.

Results

Combined therapy with laser and endoluminal iridium radiation leads to necrosis of the endoluminal portion of the tumor stenosis. Restitution of the lumen can be achieved in almost all cases. In isolated cases, following treatment, tumor tissue may no longer be detected endoscopically and histologically (Fig. **1, 2**). However, this does not mean eradication of the tumor.

Bader et al. (1) have reported their preliminary results on 40 inoperable patients with stenosis due to carcinoma of the esophagus or the cardia. The investigators achieved long-term relief of dysphagia in 80% of their patients and observed recurrent stenosis in only 20%. They conclude from their experience that the application of endoluminal iridium radiation prolongs the effect of laser treatment. Indeed, Bader et al's results compare favorably with earlier studies on laser treat-

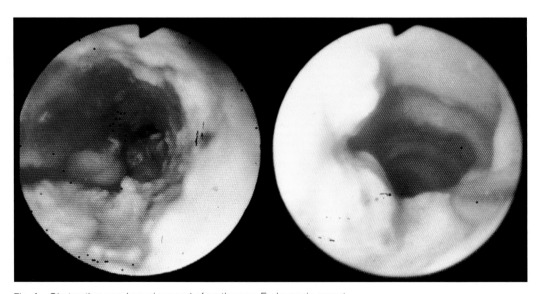

Fig. **1**   Obstructing esophageal cancer before therapy. Endoscopic aspect.

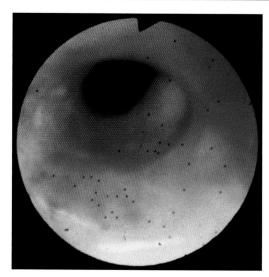

Fig. 2 Esophageal cancer 6 weeks after radiation with laser and iridium 192 (same patient as Figure 1). Optimal result with disappearance of tumor tissue and obstruction.

ment alone, which is always followed by recurrent stenosis. The complication rate in Bader et al's study was 10% (2 fistulas and 2 hemorrhages in 40 patients); the mortality was 5%. These complication rates are acceptable for a disease of such severity and poor prognosis.

Preliminary Comparison: Laser Therapy versus Laser and Endoluminal Iridium Radiation

Bader et al's (1) good results stimulated us to perform a prospective randomized comparison between laser therapy and the combination therapy with laser and endoluminal radiation with iridium-192.

In this study, patients with inoperable obstructive carcinoma of the esophagus and the cardia were included. Excluded were patients with esophagobronchial fistula and patients without detectable metastases and an endoluminal tumor extension smaller than 2 cm.

Group A received laser treatment with laser applications at 2-day intervals until a free passage was achieved. In case of recurrent stenosis, this treatment was repeated. Group B received the same initial laser treatment. In addition, they received three sessions of endoluminal radiation with iridium-192 at

1 week intervals. At each session, a dose of 7 Gy was administered at a depth of 1 cm from the radiation source. In case of recurrent stenosis, up to three further iridium radiations are applied.

The following parameters are compared in both treatment groups: Survival time, complications, frequency of recurrent stenosis, duration of intervals without dysphagia, hospitalization time, number of endoscopic procedures.

Until now, 25 patients have been enrolled in the study. Fifteen of these patients have died. Thus, the preliminary evaluation is restricted to those patients (Table 1). In group A (laser) the median survival time was 86 days compared with 120 days in group B (laser and iridium radiation). Recurrent stenosis occurred in all patients. Some patients experienced two or more recurrences. The median duration of the time period without dysphagia was longer (71 days) in the combined laser plus iridium therapy group than laser therapy alone (56 days). Patients of group A were hospitalized for 42 days, patients in group B for 24 days (median).

Esophagobronchial fistula occurred in three patients of group A and in two patients of group B. Four fistulas were treated with esophageal endoprostheses: one was treated conservatively. After the iridium radiation, three patients developed radiation esophagitis with heartburn. No death occurred related to the therapy.

These preliminary data do not confirm completly the optimistic results of Bader et al. (1) In contrast to their results with 80% long-term relief of dysphagia, all of our patients have experienced recurrent stenosis. However, our results indicate an trend in favor of prolongation of the dysphagia-free interval by the combination of the laser treatment with an endoluminal radiation with iridium-192.

It is possible that the results of combined therapy with laser and endoluminal iridium radiation could be further improved by the additional application of either external radiotherapy or chemotherapy. For the purpose of the ongoing study, we have refrained from the addition of other therapeutic modalities, because this would complicate the interpretation of the study results. This study shall be continued until a total of 60 patients are included.

	Laser	Laser + Iridium-192
Enrolled patients (n = 25)		
Sex (M/F)	9/4	8/4
Squamous cell carcinoma	5	5
Adenocarcinoma	8	7
Total recurrent stenoses	20	19
Interval between therapy and restenosis (days, mean)	26.5 (15–64)	33 (16–190)
Endoscopic procedures per patient (mean)	6.5 (3–10)	8 (4–12)
Dysphagia-free interval (day, mean)	56 (5–169)	71 (8–179)
Complications: Fistula	3	3
Esophagitis	0	3
Therapy-related mortality	0	0
Dead patients – completed follow-up (n = 15)		
Patients	8	7
Survival time (days, mean)	86 (53–191)	120 (24–208)
Hospitalization time (days, mean)	42 (13–59)	24 (9–51)

Table **1**   Results of Laser and Endoluminal Iridium-192 Radiation for Carcinomas of the Esophagus and the Cardia

Summary

The combination of laser with endoluminal iridum-192 radiation for the palliation of cancers of the esophagus and the cardia has been introduced to overcome the short-lasting effect of only laser treatment. Concluding from early experience, this method seems to prolong the effect of laser treatment alone, with a low risk of complications. However, the initial optimistic results, claiming a permanent relief of dysphagia in 80% of the patients, cannot be reproduced under prospective conditions. The combination of laser and iridium-192 radiation with other palliative methods, such as external radiation or chemotherapy, is feasible and remains to be studied in a comparative way.

References

1. Bader M, Dissler HJ, Ries G, Ultsch B, Lehr L, Siewert JR: Endokavitäre Strahlentherapie in Afterloading-Technik bei malignen Stenosen des oberen Gastrointestinaltraktes und der Gallenwege. Leber Magen Darm 15: 247–255, 1985
2. Sander R, Poesl H, Spukler A: Therapie gastrointestinaler Tumoren mit Laser. Internist 26: 22–28, 1985
3. Tytgat GN, Bartelsman JF, den Hartog Jager FC, Huibregtse K: Upper intestinal and biliary tract endoprosthesis. Dig Dis Sci 31 (Suppl. 9): 57S–76S, 1986

Laser Versus Endoprosthesis

G. N. J. Tytgat, E. M. H. Mathus-Vliegen, and F. C. A. Den Hartog Jager

Valid prospective controlled studies comparing laser and endoprosthesis for final palliation in upper intestinal cancer are nonexistent. Current views can therefore only be given in a rather descriptive fashion, stressing the possibilities, limitations, and overall results with both therapeutic modalities.

Palliation of Dysphagia with a Prosthesis

Indications and Technical Considerations

The indications, selection of material, and technical details of inserting a prosthesis have been published extensively over the last few years (10–12).

Although the number and types of commercially available tubes and insertion devices is constantly increasing, one has the impression that there is an increasing number of situations in which such tubes fail to solve the problem and in which one has to resort to homemade tygon prostheses. Tygon tubes may be necessary in perhaps one in five patients because they allow adaptation of the tube to the individual anatomy with enlarged funnels, extra retainer rings, or addition of a metal coil to strengthen the tube in case of kinking (10–12) (Fig. 1).

The same holds true for the introducing devices. Sometimes, only a specially designed metal introducer appears appropriate. The stiffness and straightness of the distal part of the introducer can gradually be enhanced, which facilitates bypassing excessively angulated stenoses (Fig. 2).

The most important and dangerous step in the procedure is the dilation of the narrowed segment. One should carefully look for the original lumen to introduce the guide wire. Most commonly used for dilation is the Savary and Eder/Puestow system. Experience with balloon dilation is limited, but this technique is also feasible (9).

The insertion of a prosthesis is for many patients still the fastest and simplest way for ultimate palliation of malignant dysphagia. Straight, even quite long cancers are usually rather easily bypassed. Not only the primary lesion, but also narrowed areas due to metastatic lymph node compression must be bypassed, which may sometimes require a tube of unusual length.

A major indication for a prosthesis is impending fistula formation. A definite malignant fistula can only be palliated with a prosthesis. No other technique except a prosthesis

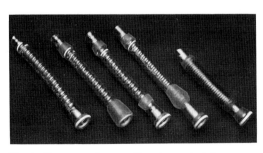

Fig. 1 Tygon prostheses with various adaptations.

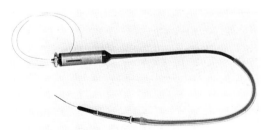

Fig. 2 Specially designed introducer, slid over a guide wire. The introducer carries a prosthesis and a pusher tube.

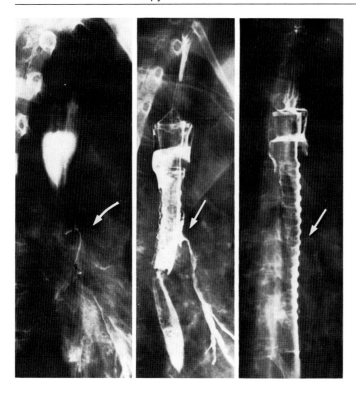

Fig. **3**   Malignant fistula, not sufficiently sealed with a standard prosthesis but fully blocked with a tube with a wide proximal ring.

can palliate the incessant coughing and aspiration of saliva. Often, a very wide funnel or extra widening is necessary to obtain full occlusion of the fistula, which may require individual adaptation of the stent (Fig. **3**). A recent alternative consists of adding a balloon around the prosthesis in order to block fully the entrance to the fistulous tract (6). A prosthesis can also be used in case of angulated lesions in the presence of a hiatal hernia, in cancer of the cardia, and in cancer of the stomach. However, bypassing extensive tumor masses in the distal or entire stomach is often technically difficult.

Limits and Problems of Stenting

Severe angulation, especially at the cardia, often leads to kinking. This can usually be corrected after strengthening the tube with a metal coil. However, the insertion of such more rigid prostheses is occasionally more difficult.

Partial occlusion of the funnel may occur when the position of a tube is excessively transverse. An extra ring may keep the funnel more in line with the esophageal axis.

Large fistulas without enough luminal narrowing to anchor the prosthesis can only be sealed after adding extra wide rings onto the tube, corresponding to the opening of the fistulous tract. Commonly, commercially available tubes fail to seal large malignant fistulas, whereas correction is possible when using prostheses with a widened funnel end.

Tube adaptation is also necessary when there is intramural tumoral extension above the narrowed area, which may lead to rapid overgrowing of the prosthesis. An extra ring or a conical proximal widening may keep the funnel edge well above the invaded, but not narrowed, segment. Intubation of multiangulated lesions remains virtually impossible, even if one succeeds in dilating such lesions with endoscopically directed balloons. Unfortunately, multiangulation is also an unfavorable condition for safe laser application. Usually, only a small feeding tube can be inserted in these often (pre)terminal patients.

Inserting a prosthesis carries appreciable morbidity and mortality rates (Table **1**). The most important complications are perforation, pressure necrosis, early and late dislocation,

Table **1**   Prosthesis for Obstructing Upper Intestinal Cancer

Initial success (absent dysphagia for solids)	90–95%
Complications: early	
Perforation	5–8%
Hemorrhage	1%
Dislocation < 4 W	15%
Complications: late	
Dislocation > 4 W	8%
Obstruction	6%
Pressure necrosis	3%
Procedure related mortality	2–4%

early and late obstruction due to food, or to overgrowing tumor, and, rather rarely, reflux esophagitis and subsequent stricturing.

Perforation is the most important complication. The incidence of perforation used to be about 8% but is now steadily decreasing to about 5%. Provided a perforation is recognized immediately, it does not drastically worsen the overall prognosis, it does, however, prolong the hospitalization. Perforation usually occurs during the dilation itself or because of a tearing action during the insertion of the prosthesis.

Palliation of Dysphagia with Laser

Indications and Technical Consideration

Some essential features of neodymium:yttrium-aluminum-garnet (Nd:YAG) application for recanalization of upper intestinal malignancy, as derived from the literature, are as follows:

– The average power setting is usually 70 W.
– Most often a 0.4 mm quartz fiber is used.
– The laser energy is usually given in 1 to 2 s pulses, form an average distance of about 1 cm from the target lesion.
– Coaxial gas flow to protect the tip is often used.
– The average number of treatment sessions is three, usually given with an interval of at least 48 hours, often longer.
– The average energy per session is approximately 5000 J.
– There is widespread variation of the total energy applied, which is, however, not

equal to the total energy that is absorbed by the tissues.

YAG laser destruction of cancerous tissue is most rewarding and easy in highly vascularized exophytic, rather straight, not too extended cancers. Malignant meniscus-type lesions are somewhat more difficult to treat, since a large portion of the cancer is intramural. Entirely submucosally spreading lesions are most difficult to treat.

YAG laser application is especially indicated in those circumstances for which a prosthesis is less appropriate, such as complete luminal obstruction, noncircumferential tumorous involvement, or the presence of a polypoid tumorous mass, not capable of anchoring a prosthesis (Fig. **4**).

Further equally important indications for laser consist of excessively soft fleshy lesions with poor anchoring capabilities, recurrences after surgical resection, lesions with 2 cm of the proximal sphincter, although this is much more difficult to treat, excessively necrotic chronically bleeding tumors with poor anchoring capabilities, inadequately functioning horizontally placed prostheses in the cardia leading to pressure necrosis by the funnel edge, and, finally, tumor spread overgrowing and obstructing a prosthesis.

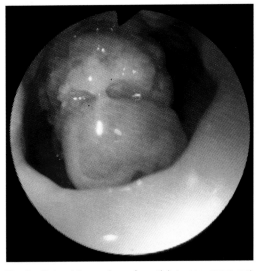

Fig. **4**   Polypoid noncircumferential tumor mass not capable of anchoring a prosthesis.

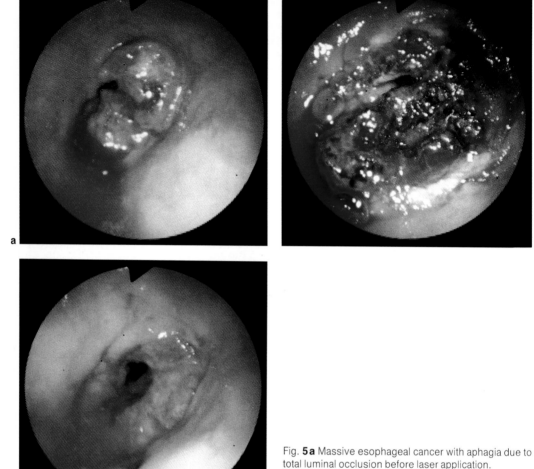

Fig. **5a** Massive esophageal cancer with aphagia due to total luminal occlusion before laser application.
b Immediately after laser application with black charring.
c Appearance after sloughing of the necrosis and partial reopening of the lumen.

The technique of laser application has been extensively reviewed lately (1–3, 5).

If at all possible, laser photocoagulation should start from below, if necessary after prior dilation of the malignant narrowing and continued while slowly withdrawing the endoscope (8). Starting from below is, however, not always possible (Fig. **5**). If laser application is repeated within 2 to 3 days after the previous session, then the yellowish-white necrotic material should be removed first. It often suffices to dislodge and remove the necrotic slough with the endoscope until viable, often slightly hemorrhagic, tumorous tissue becomes visible.

Limits and Contraindications

Factors that predict a good prognosis are a midesophageal location, a straight segment, extent less than 5 cm, an exophytic growth pattern, and an overall favorable general condition. Factors that predict a poor prognosis are a cervical location, a fixed segment, a rather horizontal segment at the cardia, a very long or tortuous lesion, submucosally spreading tumor, and an overall poor general condition.

Obvious contraindications for laser application are the presence of a fistula, a diffuse subepithelially spreading malignancy, excessively angulated lesions, and the occurrence of aiming difficulties. Excessively pronounced vascular and respiratory movements can be very disturbing. The necessity of repetitive sessions is disadvantageous. The risk of perforation and fistula formation is not negligible. Some patients complain of a retrosternal burning sensation and of distension due to gas insufflation. Transient swelling of the irradiated area may temporarily aggravate the dysphagia.

Overall Results and Discussion

A compilation of the average results as can be obtained with a prosthesis is given in Table **1**, whereas a compilation of the average results that can be obtained with YAG laser photocoagulation is given in Table **2** (4, 5, 7). As can be derived from these two tables, the relief of dysphagia is about equal for the two methods, or perhaps somewhat better with a prosthesis, provided the latter is not longer than 20 cm. Reduction in cancer load is obviously only possible with laser. The overall procedure-related mortality is presumably somewhat higher for a prosthesis. The frequency of complications is probably roughly equal for both techniques. The main disadvantage of laser photocoagulation is early restenosis requiring repetitive therapy. Occlusion of a malignant fistulous tract is only possible with a prosthesis. Highly located, multiangulated lesion or complete malignant luminal stenosis is vir-

tually only amenable to laser therapy, but also in these circumstances laser application may be difficult. The overall costs are obviously less for a prosthesis, and also the duration of hospitalization is, in general, shorter for inserting a prosthesis, compared with laser.

Based on these considerations, it appears that for several patients a tube is still the preferable definite ultimate palliation, with laser being reserved for those situations in which a tube is less satisfactory. Ideally, however, one has both techniques available. Moreover, combinations of both modalities, usually starting with laser recanalization followed by intubation, will increasingly be used in the future. There is, however, a suspicion that the risk of perforation during intubation is enhanced after prior laser therapy. Some clinicians, therefore, believe that combination therapy may prove helpful provided intubation is performed before the esophagus is rendered inelastic by laser-induced fibrosis.

Does intubation or laser vaporization benefit the patient? The answer is yes insofar as the dysphagia is eliminated in the vast majority of the patients. However, carefully conducted quality of life studies, comparing various palliative approaches, have not been carried out and are awaited, but such studies will be difficult to perform.

Table **2** Nd:YAG Laser for Obstructing Upper Intestinal Cancer

	No.	%
Initial success (absent dysphagia for solids)		75–85
Laser sessions	~ 3 (2–6)	
Bougienage sessions	1–5	
Complications		
Perforation		~ 4–5
Fistulas		~ 1
Hemorrhage		~ 1
Sepis		0.5–1
Procedure-related mortality		1–2
Dysphagia-free interval 3–6 W		~ 60–70
> 3 MS		20–25

References

1. Bown SG: Endoscopic laser therapy for oesophageal cancer. Endoscopy 18 (Suppl 13):26–31, 1986
2. Bown SG, Matthewson K, Swain CP, Clark CG: Follow-up of laser palliation for malignant dysphagia. Gut 26:114, 1985
3. Ell C, Hochberger J, Lux G: Clinical experience of non-contact and contact Nd: YAG laser therapy in inoperable tumour stenoses of the oesophagus and stomach. Laser Med Sci 1:143, 1986
4. Fleischer D, Kessler F, Haye O: Endoscopic Nd: YAG laser therapy for carcinoma of the esophagus: A new palliative approach. Am J Surg 143:280–283, 1982
5. Fleischer D, Sivak MV: Endoscopic Nd: YAG laser therapy as a palliation for esophagogastric cancer. Gastroenterology 89:827, 1985
6. Lux G, Wilson D, Wilson J, Demling L: A cuffed tube for the treatment of esophagobronchial fistulae. Endoscopy 19:28–30, 1987
7. Mathus-Vliegen EMH, Tytgat GNJ: Laser photocoagulation in the palliative treatment of upper digestive tract tumors. Cancer 57:396–399, 1986

8. Riemann JF, Ell CH, Lux G, Demling L: Combined therapy of malignant stenoses of the upper gastrointestinal tract by means of laser beam and bougienage. Endoscopy 17:43–48, 1985

9. Tytgat GNJ: Dilatation therapy of benign esophageal stenoses. World J Surg (1987)

10. Tytgat GNJ, Bartelsman JFWM, den Hartog Jager FCA, Huibregtse K: Upper intestinal and biliary tract endoprosthesis. Dig Dis Sci 31:57S–76S, 1986

11. Tytgat GNJ, den Hartog Jager FCA, Bartelsman JFWM: Endoscopic prosthesis for advanced esophageal cancer. Endoscopy 18: (Suppl 3) 32–39, 1986

12. Tytgat GNJ, Huibregtse K, Bartelsman JFWM, den Hartog Jager FCA: Endoscopic palliative therapy of gastrointestinal and biliary tumors with prostheses. Clin Gastroenterol 15:249, 1986

Laser in Combination with Radiotherapy and Chemotherapy

R. Lambert, J. C. Souquet, A. Chavaillon, and F. Descos

The photodestruction of tumors with laser radiation is currently performed in the digestive tract in monotherapy. The local destruction of the tumor (complete or partial) is achieved without resection. On the other hand, laser therapy may be included in a multimodal protocol when extensive tumoral destruction requires addition, or potentiation, of different procedures, such as chemotherapy. The respective choice between laser in monotherapy or laser in combination is made after considering surgery as an alternative and analyzing the characteristics of the tumor.

Objective of Treatment and the Surgical Alternative

A nonsurgical protocol is adopted only after careful analysis of the efficacy, morbidity, and mortality of surgery (palliative or curative exeresis) versus the patient's health condition.

Simple palliation of symptoms without prolonging life requires a *partial destruction* of the tumor, that is, of the part obstructing the digestive lumen. It is proposed to patients in a very poor condition, with advanced cancer. There is no surgical alternative; therefore laser photodestruction is proposed in monotherapy.

When, in addition to palliation of symptoms, a delayed evolution of the tumor (and a prolonged life span) is desirable, the treatment requires *subtotal destruction* of the malignant tissue, including its intramural basis. To this purpose, laser photodestruction is often combined with other procedures. This also concerns tumors with regional lymph node invasion. A multimodal protocol is proposed for patients with advanced cancer when the health condition is maintained. The alternative to be considered is palliative surgical excision.

Curative therapy is proposed when there is sound evidence that *complete destruction* of the malignant tissue is possible. This concerns either benign tumors, or cancer. In the latter condition, the pattern at endoscopy must indicate a superficial tumor; of course, at the preoperative stage, a possible extension of the cancer in the muscularis propria (false superficial type of tumor) or in regional lymph nodes cannot be excluded. This is why multimodal, nonsurgical treatment is often required for the superficial type of cancer. The surgical alternative is of course, a curative exeresis.

Characteristics of the Tumor

Adoption of a multimodal, nonsurgical protocol is also based on the characteristics of the tumor: its respective susceptibility to destruction through laser, chemotherapy, or radiotherapy; its tendency to regional and distant propagation; its evolutive pattern, including the overall 5-year survival rate and the specific rates with treatment.

In the *esophagus*, the squamous cell cancer fullfils most of the criteria in favor of a multimodal, nonsurgical protocol. It will be selected as a model in this text.

In the *stomach*, the adenocarcinoma tumor is usually treated by surgical resection. Indications for a nonsurgical protocol are very limited. Indeed, the tumor susceptibility to cytostatic agents or radiation is poor and laser photodestruction is usually performed in monotherapy, the two respective indications being palliation of dysphagia in tumors obstructing the cardia, and attempt to complete tumor destruction in superficial cancer when the operative contraindication is evident.

In the *colon and rectum*, the adenocarcinoma at an advanced stage is usually treated by surgery. If a nonsurgical protocol is adopted for palliation, there is no definite advantage in combining agents; therefore, laser photodestruction is used in monotherapy, palliation of symptoms being the objective. On the other hand, most cases of superficial cancer are identical to intramucosal cancer foci in adenomatous polyps. They are adequately treated in monotherapy either by diathermic snare (resection) or laser photodestruction (10% of cases). There is no place for a multimodal protocol in such lesions.

Decision Analysis in Squamous Cell Cancer of the Esophagus

Elements of treatment in a patient with squamous cell cancer of the esophagus include recanalization of the esophageal lumen through dilation, stent, or laser photodestruction; chemotherapy; radiotherapy; palliative or curative exeresis. The decision depends on symptoms, the physical condition of the patient, and tumor staging. The overall prognosis of the disease is very poor; this is related to the rapid regional spreading of the tumor in the lymphatic system and to a tendency for distant metastases even when the local destruction of the tumor is total (2). The global 5-year survival rate in surgical series is not much different from data in cancer registries, including all untreated cases. However a considerable progress has been made in two directions. First, a much better prognosis is found in patients with small tumors, limited to the esophageal wall when the lymph nodes are negative. Surgery is therefore the treatment of choice for a patient in good health, still young, when the preoperative staging indicates a limited tumor and an abscence of lymphatic extension. However, this concerns a very small percentage of the symptomatic patients. Second, the short-term prognosis (survival rate at 1 year and at 2 year) has been improved in all groups of patients and of treatment (surgical or nonsurgical). The progress results mainly from the control of dysphagia.

Symptoms

Dysphagia is the basic symptom in esophageal cancer, resulting in weight loss and malnutrition. In the absence of surgical excision, the reestablishment of the esophageal lumen improves the patient's condition immediately. The weight curve is stabilized or returns to a positive slope. This can be achieved by laser recanalization or stenting. The best results from laser treatment are achieved when the obstructive tumor is noncircumferential and

exophytic rather than infiltrative; in such patients, the symptom relief is prolonged and laser sessions are required at long intervals. On the other hand, an infiltrant and stenotic tumor requires stenting. Laser treatment of such circumferential lesions induces, indeed, a prompt recurrence of the stenosis through inflammation and fibrosis, the relief of dysphagia being transient. Of course, the presence of a neoplastic esophagobronchial fistula also requires a stent.

Patients with a superficial endoscopic type of esophageal cancer have *no dysphagia,* and may even demonstrate no symptoms indicating esophageal disease; therefore, the treatment is not concerned with symptom relief and its objective is limited to tumor destruction.

Health Status of the Patient

In assessing operability, age is considered an important risk factor. The rate of mortality after thoracic esophagectomy is too high in patients more than 70 years old, therefore, they should seldom be considered for surgery. Associated and epidemiologically correlated cancers are common in such patients; they are either antecedent and previously cured, or in simultaneous evolution. They are located especially in the oropharynx or the larynx. Their presence is a strong argument in favor of nonsurgical treatment. In alcoholic patients esophageal squamous cell cancer is often associated to other visceral diseases, such as liver cirrhosis, chronic emphysema, cardiomyopathy. When at an advanced stage of development, they require nonsurgical treatment.

Preoperative Staging of the Tumor

Preoperative staging of the tumor is not identical to the preoperative determination of operability. The morphologic classification of the tumor concerning the depth of invasion in the esophageal wall, in periesophageal tissues and the status of regional lymph nodes should approach the data usually obtained on the postoperative specimen (pTNM, staging). The procedures for staging the esophageal tumor include: *endoscopy,* analysis of the endoluminal surface of the tumor; *echoendoscopy,* analysis of the tumoral extension in the muscularis propria of the esophagus and of the mediastinal lymph nodes; *computed tomogra-*

phy scan; and *bronchoscopy.* The preoperative staging includes also exploration for distant malignant lymph nodes and distant metastases.

The cancer is classified as superficial at endoscopy when the tumor surface is slightly altered: either flat, elevated, depressed, or with a mixed pattern. Esophageal peristalsis is maintained. However, an echoendoscopy is required to separate the superficial cancer (tumor invasion limited to the mucosa and submucosa) from the false superficial cancer (extension of the tumor across the muscularis propria). Concerning this specific point, the accuracy of the procedure is more than 90%. Lower figures characterize the screening of mediastinal lymph nodes as malignant or benign. An exophytic, polypoid, nonulcerated tumor is an uncommon finding in the esophagus. Despite its obstructive character, it may correspond to a superficial cancer (elevated type), after staging.

The cancer is classified as advanced at endoscopy when there is endoluminal obstruction combined with vegetations, ulcer, and infiltration. The preoperative staging by echoendoscopy is incomplete when the tube stops at the upper pole of the stenosis (around 40% of cases). Taking all elements into account, the tumor will be classified as localized to the esophageal wall (no propagation in the mediastinum) or extra esophageal. The regional extension of the tumor includes mediastinal invasion, adhesion to aorta or pericardum, bronchial invasion, and possibly bronchial fistula. Malignant mediastinal and celiac lymph nodes are also explored and classified.

Laser in Mono- versus Multimodal, Nonsurgical Therapy

Laser in Monotherapy

Laser will achieve recanalization of the esophageal lumen in a single, or a few repeated sessions, in the presence of obstructive vegetations. However, maintenance of a large lumen requires repeated sessions at intervals from 4 to 6 weeks: there is a rapid regrowth of the tumor combined with inflammation and fibrosis induced by the thermal burn. Therefore, the tumor morphology progressively alters to a narrow, inextensible, channel, requiring dilation (more and more difficult) rather

than laser destruction. The symptomatic relief is usually good during the first 3 months of follow-up. Later, complications may occur (mediastinal or bronchial perforation during dilation) or stenting may be necessary. The life span of such patients, usually limited to 6 months, is more than 1 year in only 10% of cases. Laser in monotherapy is preferable to esophageal stenting in most cases of palliation, but its indications are restricted to patients in a very poor condition when all other procedures are contraindicated.

Laser in a Multimodal Protocol

Multimodal therapy is proposed on the following bases (11, 12). First, the prompt relief of dysphagia is the primary request of the patient, and laser photodestruction is the best procedure to obtain this result. Therefore, it should be included at the initial stage of the treatment: later there is no need for repeated laser sessions if the luminal patency is maintained by other long-acting procedures. Second, recent progress in oncology is associated with multimodal protocols. Different cytotoxic agents, acting through different means on malignant cells (chemotherapy, radiotherapy), will show cumulative effects either with a simple addition, or with potentiation. Of course, the cumulative character concerns not only the antitumoral activity, but also the side effects; therefore, increased caution is required during the surveillance program.

The results of multimodal protocols conducted in patients with esophageal cancer are found in a number of publications made available during the last 5 years. They concern either the combination of various cytotoxic agents or their association with radiotherapy. Reports on *curative radiotherapy* stress that despite a high response rate of the tumor, the long-term result is poor due to a high toll of local recurrences and distant metastases (about 50% for both). A number of *cytostatic agents* have been on trial; their efficacy in squamous cell cancer with a positive tumoral response is admitted for 5-fluorouracil, bleomycin, mitomycin, cisplatin, methotrexate, doxorubicin, vindesine. As a matter of fact, the best association is between 5-fluorouracil and cisplatin when efficacy is considered in relation to toxicity. Programs combining cytostatic and radiotherapy have been proposed in two different conditions: either as nonsurgical multimodal protocols in nonoperable patients, or as adjuvant preoperative (neoadjuvant), or possible postoperative programs in patients undergoing thoracic esophagectomy.

In patients with *inoperable esophageal cancer,* the association of cytostatic agents and radiotherapy has a number of advantages, stressed by Kolaric (10): the response rate of the tumor is high (more than 50%), the proportion of complete responses with negative biopsies at the site of the lesion reaches 40% in some protocols, the toxicity is decreased due to the longer duration of the protocol, the duration of the remission is acceptable, varying from 6 to 18 months. Of course, although the short-term morbidity is improved, there is still no clear demonstration of prolonged survival.

In patients undergoing a *thoracic esophagectomy,* the preliminary results of neoadjuvant chemotherapy or radiotherapy are encouraging. A number of investigational trials (1, 3–10, 15–18) indicate an increased rate of resectability and an absence of residual disease in the resected esophagus in up to 30% of cases. However, the operative mortality increases to a prohibitive level in some protocols. This is why the available data do not yet support the routine application of such protocols before (or after) surgery: they remain on trial for a few years more. Examples are the respective data reported in 1984 (14) and 1987 (13) by the teams of the Wayne State School of Medicine and the Detroit Medical Center. In the initial trial (14) surgical excision was assumed to be the main step; neoadjuvant therapy called for 5-fluorouracil, cisplatin, and radiotherapy. The median survival in this group reached 18 months. Long-term survivors were found only in patients (25%) who had no residual cancer on the operative specimen. However, the curative efficacy of surgery was in question because the same patients died later (30 to 60 months) from distant metastases, whereas the patients with residual cancer on the operative specimen died early from this disease. The second trial (13) excluded the surgical step; the median survival of this group was longer (22 months) and the quality of life was improved. Only four patients were submitted to delayed surgery when the failure of the nonsurgical protocol was evident.

In summary, the multimodal protocol widely accepted, improves the quality of life in those patients not feasible for surgery. This is now an acceptable alternative to surgical treatment. On the other hand, the benefit of chemotherapy and radiotherapy as an adjuvant to surgical treatment is not demonstrated in advanced cancer. Furthermore, the efficacy of surgery as a curative treatment is questionable in such patients. Of course, for the minority of patients with superficial cancer, especially an intraepithelial tumor with negative lymph nodes, the curative value of surgery has been proved by long-term results.

The rationale for including thermal laser, that is, neodymium:yttrium-aluminum-garnet (Nd:YAG), treatment in al multimodal protocol is the cumulative effect on tumor destruction; laser is well adapted to reduce the volume of the endoluminal protruding part of the tumor. The amount of malignant tissue submitted to radiotherapy should be as small as possible to enhance the efficacy of this procedure. The laser session will be introduced at the first stage of the protocol, resulting in prompt relief of dysphagia. It follows, however, the first chemotherapy session, the pretreated tumor being more susceptible to thermal destruction. After this therapeutic step, there is no room for repeated laser sessions. When a nonthermal laser treatment (photodynamic therapy) is selected, it is aimed at selective destruction of a superficial cancer and is performed in monotherapy. Multimodal therapy can then only be proposed 2 months later to avoid additive toxic photosensitization side effects.

Our Experience in Lyon

Selection of Therapeutic Programs

From August 1981 to August 1987, 400 patients with squamous cell cancer in the esophagus entered a nonsurgical therapeutic program, including laser. When such a program is selected, a delayed alteration of the management and surgical treatment occurs if the control of symptoms and disease is inadequate and if there is no operative contraindication; this occurs in approximately 5% of cases. *Advanced cancer* was present in 85%, of which 30% were treated by the Nd:YAG thermal laser in monotherapy for simple palliation and 55% were treated according to a multimodal protocol, including chemotherapy sessions (5-fluorouracil, cisplatin), NG:YAG laser, and radiotherapy. An endoscopic pattern of *superficial cancer* occurred in approximately 15% of patients (i.e., 56 cases). In this group, most laser treatments were performed with the nonthermal procedure. Furthermore, 40% were treated in monotherapy and 60% in a multimodal protocol.

During the same period, 166 other patients with the same disease were examined at diagnostic endoscopy, and the decision for treatment was not made by the same group and laser treatment was not proposed. In this diagnostic group, the relative rate of superficial versus advanced cancer (endoscopic pattern) was 6.0% (10 cases of superficial cancer).

Results

In advanced cancer (laser in monotherapy) a symptomatic relief can be achieved for 3 to 6 months. Later, degradation of the patient's condition occurs and the survival rate over 1 year is about 10%. Laser sessions are repeated at regular intervals and delayed stent positioning is eventually required (infiltrant stenosis, or fistula).

In advanced cancer, (laser in multimodal protocol) a long-term relief of dysphagia is expected without repetition of the laser sessions. Dilation in the course of follow-up may be required if the esophageal scar is stenotic. Usually, the weight of the patient increases during treatment and the nutritional status is maintained. The survival rate depends on: (1) the evolution of the tumor, complete or partial response, recurrence at the local or regional level, distant metastases (liver, lung, brain); and (2) the evolution of associated diseases or correlated cancers. Therefore, the mortality is unrelated to the treated cancer in approximately 50% of cases. The survival rate, linked to the evolution of the squamous cell cancer, is about 70% at 1 year and 50% at 2 years. Of course, crude data, including the other causes of mortality, are lower.

In superficial cancer (endoscopic pattern), laser is used either in monotherapy or in a multimodal protocol. The influence of the treatment on symptoms is slight, since dysphagia is usually absent; on the other hand, the health condition of the patient usually improves. As in the other group, survival de-pends on the evolution of cancer and of associated diseases. The survival rate linked to the evolution of cancer only is about 85% at 1 year and 75% at 2 years. Mortality correlated to cancer is mainly from distant metastases. After 12 to 48 months, a recurrent cancer often develops in the esophagus, and can be adequately treated in monotherapy by laser.

The 56 patients entering a nonsurgical protocol in our experience had a mean age of 66 years, a severe associated disease was present in 27, an associated (previous or simultaneous) cancer in 16, and liver metastases in 5. They were classified as superficial from their endoscopic pattern. From the endosonographic staging, it is estimated that 40% were actually false superficial tumors. The respective ratio of mono- versus multimodal laser therapy was 50:50 in this group. The global survival rate including all causes of mortality was 72% at 1 year, and 47% at 2 years. The mortality rate unrelated to cancer was 57%.

Nonsurgical Multimodal Protocols, Including Laser

The inclusion of a patient in a multimodal laser protocol is based on two assumptions: surgical treatment is contraindicated and the patient is able to receive treatment by cytostatic agents and radiotherapy. The main contraindication to chemotherapy is correlated to the hyperhydration protocol. Therefore, extreme caution is advised in elderly patients (more than 75 years old) or those with severe cardiovascular deficiency.

Advanced Cancer
Basic Protocol

1. The elements of treatment include chemotherapy sessions for 4 days, with the following agents in continuous infusion and rehydration: 5-fluorouracil, 1000 mg/m^2/day for 4 days, cisplatin, 80 mg/m^2/day for 4 days, Nd:YAG laser thermal abrasion of the protruding part of the tumor. Radiotherapy is in a split protocol, including ten 3 Gy sessions in 2 weeks and five 3 Gy sessions in 1 week. Treatment, by preference, is with a linear (18–25 MeV) accelerator.

2. The chronology of the treatment is shown in Table **1**. The *first stage* includes chemotherapy followed by laser photodestruction. The *second stage* includes radiotherapy

Table **1**   Nonsurgical Multimodal Protocol of Treatment in Squamous Cell Cancer of the Esophagus Protocol for the First 6 Months

Week 1	Day 1–4	First chemotherapy session 5-fluorouracil, 1000 mg/m^2/ day, 4 days Cisplatin 80 mg/m^2, 1 day
	Day 5	Nd:YAG laser, first session (abrasion of the tumor)
	Day 7	Nd:YAG laser, second session
Week 2–3	–	–
Week 4	Day 1–4	Second chemotherapy session
	Day 1–5	Radiotherapy, 3 Gy/day, Linear acceleration, 18–25 MeV
Week 5	Day 1	Endoscopic examination; eventual dilation
	Day 1–5	Radiotherapy, 3 Gy/day
Week 6		Third chemotherapy session
Week 7–8	–	–
Week 9		Endoscopic examination; eventual dilation
Week 10	Day 1–5	Radiotherapy, 3 Gy/day
Week 11	–	–
Week 12–24		Endoscopic examination One to three chemotherapy sessions

combined with chemotherapy in the first part of the split protocol. The *third stage* includes the second part of the radiotherapy program. Esophageal dilations may be required during the course of the treatment to treat a stenotic scar. Altogether, this treatment takes about 3 months.

3. The symptom relief depends essentially on the tumor morphology. The best results are obtained with noncircumferential exophytic lesions. On the other hand, infiltrant and circumferential stenotic tumors usually remain with some dysphagia and require repeated dilation. This procedure (and not laser irradiation) is the possible cause of perforations in the mediastinum (nonsurgical treatment, including aspiration and antibiotics) or in the bronchial tree (stent required). Therefore, surgical treatment should be preferred in this group of patients when there is no operative contraindication.

4. Follow-up after the first 3 months includes, at a minimum: endoscopic and radiographic exploration of the esophagus, echographic exploration of the liver, and radiographs of the chest.

In the esophagus, more or less complete destruction is expected in the exophytic noncircumferential tumors. The scar is usually small, with a very slight stenosis, fibrotic aspect, and mucosal fragility to contact. Forceps biopsies are often negative. For other tumors, the destruction is often incomplete: the persisting tumor is usually infiltrated, ulcerated, and mixed with fibrosis. In some patients a chronic ulcer persists with necrosis. Later, postradiation necrosis may cause either obstruction or bronchial fistula, if the initial tumor had a large extra esophageal extension in the mediastinum. This has a bad prognosis and requires stenting. In the long run, development of metastases is common, even in patients with a normal esophagus.

5. Tolerance of treatment is usually good, and hospitalization periods are short. Many patients after the initial period of the treatment resume their professional activity for some time. Side effects or complications are observed when the contraindications to chemotherapy have not been respected. The main complications are coronary ischemia or cerebrovascular spasms. They are also observed if more than six chemotherapy sessions are performed.

Specific Protocols

According to the tumor morphology, the protocol may be altered: (1) if bronchial invasion (without perforation) is detected at the initial exploration. The first stage of the treatment is prolonged with repeated sessions of chemotherapy. The second stage (radiotherapy) is performed only if a response of the bronchial tumor is observed with a return to normal. This procedure avoids most of the radiation-induced fistulas. (2) If the primary tumor is accompanied by numerous tumoral foci, at distance in the esophgagus (stressing an extensive lymphatic propagation); emphasis should also be placed on chemotherapy with repeated sessions before radiotherapy. Usually the esophageal lumen returns to normal. After a 6 to 18 month period of remission, the cancer is located in the cervical esophagus, invading the upper sphincter, the symptomatic relief is usually poor. Indeed the tumor is often infiltrant and the nervous control of swallowing is often altered. Therefore, in such patients, the management is improved by percutaneous gastrostomy. It may be withdrawn after a few weeks, if the local evolution is favorable.

Superficial Cancer

This concerns the endoscopic pattern of the superficial cancer in the esophagus. Staging by echoendoscopy is required to separate superficial cancer (limited to the mucosa and submucosa) from the false superficial cancer, entering the muscularis propria. This distinction determines the selection of a therapeutic protocol.

False Superficial Cancer

The management of such patients is similar to advanced cancer. They have a better prognosis. Usually the esophageal lumen returns to normal with a nonstenotic scar. Cancer evolution after remission will be either from metastases or from local recurrences. The latter, usually of the superficial type, may be treated by laser in monotherapy.

Confirmed Superficial Cancer, with Distant Metastases

The management is the same as that for false superficial cancer if there is a single metastasis. If metastases are multiple, contrasting with a maintained health condition of the patient, emphasis should be placed on chemotherapy and the stage of radiotherapy is withheld.

Confirmed Superficial Cancer Without Metastases

This lesion is an elective indication for photodynamic therapy.

Therefore, the first stage of the protocol is monotherapy: injection of the hematoporphyrin derivative (2 to 3 mg/kg), irradiation at 630 nm (from 100 to 200 j/cm^2 after an interval of 2 to 3 days.

The second stage of the protocol is an observation period of 2 months, allowing clearance of the photosensitizing agent from the body; during the first month, the patient should avoid any direct exposure to the sunlight to prevent cutaneous intolerance.

The third stage of the protocol is based on radiotherapy in combination with chemotherapy (one to two sessions). During the follow-up, echoendoscopic examination of the scar is required at 3 and 6 months. Recurrences are often observed at intervals from 12 to 48 months after the initial treatment, and they are treated by photodynamic therapy without complement.

References

1. Advani SH, Saikia TK, Swaroop S, et al: Anterior chemotherapy in esophageal cancer. Cancer 56:1502–1506, 1985
2. Anderson L, Lad T: Autopsy findings in squamous cell carcinoma of the esophagus. Cancer 50:1587–1590, 1982
3. Franklin R, Steiger Z, Valshampayan G, et al: Combined modality therapy for esophageal squamous cell carcinoma. Cancer 51:1062–1071, 1983
4. Hellman S: Cancer of the esophagus: A brighter future. J Clin Oncol 2:73–74, 1984
5. Jobsen JS, Vanandel JG, Eiskenboom WH, et al: Carcinoma of the esophagus. Treatment results. Radiother Oncol 5:101–108, 1980
6. Kelsen D: Treatment of advanced esophageal cancer. Cancer 50:2576–2581, 1982
7. Kelsen D: Chemotherapy-based multi-modality therapy of esophageal cancer. In: Primary Chemotherapy in Cancer Medicine. New York: Liss, 1985 (pp 241–252)
8. Kelsen DP, Bains A, Hilaris B, et al: Combination chemotherapy of esophageal carcinoma using cisplatin, vindesine and bleomycin. Cancer 49:1174–1177, 1982
9. Kelsen, DP, Weston E, Kurtz R, et al: Squamous-cell carcinoma of the esophagus. Cancer 45:1558–1561, 1980
10. Kolaric K: Combination of cytostatics and radiation – a new trend in the treatment of inoperable esophageal cancer. In: Primary Chemotherapy in Cancer Medicine. New York: Liss, Alan 1985; 259–282
11. Lambert R: Cancer in the esophagus. Principles of laser treatment in Jensen D, JM Brunetaud (eds): Medical Laser Endoscopy. Nijhoff, Amsterdam 1987
12. Lambert R, Sabben G, Chavaillon A, et al: Nd Yag laser therapy for epidermoid cancer of the esophagus. Gastroenterology 86:1151, 1984
13. Leichman L, Herskovic CG, Leichman PB, et al: Non operative therapy for squamous cell cancer in the esophagus. J Clin Oncol 5:365–370, 1987
14. Leichman L, Steiger A, Seydel HG, et al: Preoperative chemotherapy plus radiation therapy for patients with cancer of the esophagus: Potentially curative approach. J Clin Oncol 2:75–79, 1984

15. Lokich JJ, Shea M, Chaffey J: Sequential infusional 5-fluorouracil followed by concomitant radiation for tumor of the esophagus and gastroesophageal junction. Cancer 60:275–279, 1987

16. Resbeut M, Le Prise-Fleury E, Ben-Hassel M, et al: Squamous cell carcinoma of the esophagus. Cancer 56:1246–1250, 1986

17. Schlag P, Herrmann R, Fritze D, et al: Preoperative chemotherapy in localized cancer of the esophagus with cis-platinum, vindesine and bleomycin. In: Primary Chemotherapy in Cancer Medicine. New York: Liss, 1985 (pp 253–256)

18. Steiger Z, Franklin R, Wilson RF, et al: Eradication and palliation of squamous cell carcinoma of the esophagus with chemotherapy, radiotherapy and surgical therapy. J Thorac Cardiovasc Surg 82:713–719, 1981

Future Trends

Low-Power Contact Neodymium:Yttrium-Aluminum-Garnet

C. Ell and J. Hochberger

Low-Power Contact Neodymium:Yttrium-Aluminum-Garnet Laser Therapy

At present, high-power neodymium:yttrium-aluminum-garnet (Nd:YAG) lasers of up to 100 W are used for noncontact endoscopic laser therapy in the gastrointestinal tract. A first attempt to reduce power output and, as a consequence, the costs of the laser system and therapy was done by Sabben et al. (7) in 1983. They used a naked fiber in contact with the tissue,with a laser power output of only 30 W. With the development of ceramic and metal tips at the distal end of the light guide, new forms of energy application became available (1, 10). However, as in other fields of laser medicine, clinicians have just begun to evaluate the potentials of the new contact methods. Therefore, only preliminary information and results can be presented.

Characteristics of the Contact Methods

Naked Fiber

A 600 μm fiber is used. At the distal end the Teflon coating is stripped from the fiber. The laser power output necessary for a sufficient therapeutic effect is 30 to 40 W. Higher ranges induce burning of the fiber coating. The energy can be applied to the surface of a lesion as well as interstitially in large exophytic tumor masses.

For low-power (1 to 2 W) interstitial therapy with a bare fiber, see page 129 ff.

Ceramic Probes

At present, three companies (SLT, USA; Osada, Japan; MBB, W-Germany) offer ceramic tips, made of aluminium oxide (AL_2O_3) (artificial sapphire). The probes have a high melting point (2000°C), and demonstrate a good transmission of the laser beam of about 85 to 95%. There are various shapes with different optical properties available (Fig. 1). The tips can be screwed onto a metal connector attached to the tip of the fiber. The outer diameter of the tip varies between 1.8 and 2.2 mm. To reduce adhesion to the tissue, it is recommended to install a continuous water irrigation system (water flow, 5 to 10 ml/min) (Fig. 2). Additionally, the ceramic tip and its metal shaft are cooled by the water. A special silicon sealing is necessary to protect the connection between the proximal end of the light guide and the laser resonator if tips are used with an extraneus light quide system (e.g., MBB). The required power output varies between 5 and 20 W. The tips can be used for several treatment sessions, according to our experience, between 5 to 15 times.

Metal Probes

The metal tips (Trimedyne, USA) that have come onto the market recently are recommended for single use only, a fact that raises the price of treatment. For different laser systems, varying adapters are available.

The metal probes work as a soldering iron and provoke temperatures from 300° to 1200°C (Fig. 3). Newly developed probes with a central "window" permit also the direct light transmission into the tissue so that the combi-

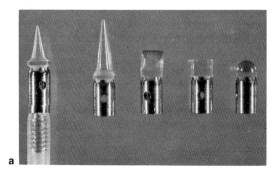

a

Endoscopic Contact Probes

Coagulation	Vaporization	Incision/Excision

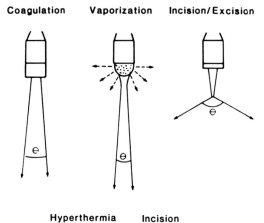

Hyperthermia Photoradiation Therapy	Incision

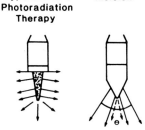

b

Fig. **1a, b** Sapphire contact tips of various shapes and different optical properties (SLT, USA).

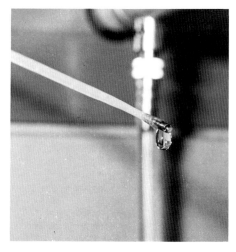

Fig. **2** Sapphire contact tip with continous water irrigation to avoid adhesion to the tissue and damage to the tip.

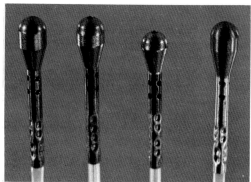

Fig. **3** Metal probes of different shape (Nytech/Trimedyne, USA).

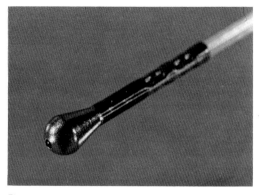

Fig. **4** Metal tip with central window (Spectraprobe 80).

nation of deep light penetration and thermal contact effect can be used therapeutically (Fig. **4**).

Experimental Studies

Only one experimental study can be found in the literature for contactlaser using a naked fiber at power settings of 20 to 40 W (7) not to be confused with low-power interstitial therapy at 1 to 2 W with long exposure times (see page 129ff). In comparison to superficial irradiation techniques normally used, Sabben et al. (7) showed that the size of an induced lesion increases when the fiber is in interstitial tissue contact. Therefore, and because the use of a naked fiber is more economical than that of the gas flow protected, teflon-coated fiber, Sabben et al. recommended the naked fiber and interstitial laser therapy.

Several experimental studies have already been published on the contact method with ceramic tips (1, 4, 8, 10, 11). Different tissue effects regarding the extension of the lesion and the relation of the coagulation to the vaporization zone can be achieved with different kinds of tips and different irradiation parameters (power output, 5 to 25 W; exposure time, 0.5 to 20.0 s). Depending on their shape, the ceramic tips work as focusing or defocusing lenses (see Fig. **1b**). Finally, when the surface of the probe adheres to the tissue or is covered by carbonated material, additional to the optical effect, there is a thermal effect of the ceramic tip similar to a soldering iron.

The metal tips, on the other hand, work exclusively as soldering irons. The available experimental studies show good potential for their use in hemostasis (4). Experimental data with regard to vaporization capacity do not exist yet. In a pilot study in rats we compared the metal with the ceramic tips and with the following results.

1. Similar effects in respect to evaporated tissue volume, achieved coagulation zone, and adhesion to tissue can be seen with 11 W "hot" tip and 14 to 16 W sapphire vaporization tip, 30 s total exposure time in 10-s steps. The development of smoke was more intense with the metal tips.
2. A disadvantage of the metal tips was the long time needed (about 5 s) to heat the probe up to red or even yellow or white hot (600° to 1200 °C). This temperature is

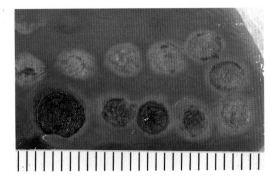

Fig. **5** Metal tip: possible tissue effects during the cooling-down phase of the tip. On the left side below contact tissue vaporisation at 11 W, 250 J total, in the following lesions in 1 s intervals without any further energy supply (scale 1 mm).

needed to achieve a sufficient vaporization effect and to prevent sticking to the tissue surface. In practice, the long heating-up time might prove too long, for example, in the therapy of bleeding ulcers with difficulties in visualizing the bleeding vessel.

3. Another disadvantage is the long time it takes for the probe to cool down after therapy (Fig. **5**). After stopping the energy application, the probe needs more than 10 s to cool down to temperatures that are neither dangerous for the surrounding tissue nor for the endoscopic equipment.

A comparison between the noncontact and the contact methods concerning the energy required for similar tissue effects appears difficult if not impossible: There are many parameters, e.g., the pressure exerted on the tissue during contact irradiation, the distance between the end of the light guide and the tissue (noncontact), the applied power and pulse duration at identical total energy, which greatly influence the tissue effect. As far as available experimental data show, the contact method requires less than one-third to one-fifth of the energy that is necessary with the noncontact method to achieve similar tissue effects (Fig. **6**) (7). For the ceramic tips, a power output of 16 to 20 W is sufficient for both vaporization and coagulation, with the hemispherical, so-called vaporization, tip.

Whether the so-called coagulation ceramic tip is more effective than the noncontact

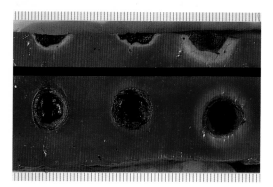

Fig. **6** Comparison of the tissue effects of different application methods. From left to right: "GI" metal tip, 11 W, 1000 J total; vaporization sapphire tip, 14 W, 1400 J total; noncontact method (NC), 5 mm irradiation distance, 80 W, 3500 J total (scale 1 mm).

method for controlling hemorrhage is uncertain; experimental data are not yet available. The various other ceramic tips (Fig. **1**) do not seem to be of much additional value in gastroenterologic laser therapy.

Clinical Experiences

Major experiences with the naked fiber obviously exist only in France (2). Recently, Naveau et al. (6) reported on a comparison between the noncontact method and the contact method with the naked fiber in 40 patients. With the interstitial technique, only half the treatment sessions were necessary compared the noncontact method (6). In our view, the interstitial technique can be recommended only for an experienced laser therapist for the treatment of large exophytic tumors, especially in the lower gastrointestinal tract. Otherwise, the risk of early or late perforation seems unjustifiably high. The naked fiber is not suited for control of gastrointestinal hemorrhage.

Whether the value of the ceramic or metal tips for hemostasis is similar to that of other contact procedures, such as electrocoagulation (electrohydrothermoprobe, heater probe), has up to now not sufficiently been reported.

Concerning tumor treatment with the contact technique using ceramic and metal tips, the first published reports claimed better results and easier handling for the contact technique compared with the noncontact method

(8, 9). Obviously, the studies were small and did not exceed 20 patients. In 1986 we reported our first experience with the contact method in 24 patients (3). Up to now we have trated 42 patients with the contact technique (132 patients with the noncontact method). From our practical experience, we can state the following respective advantages or disadvantages of the two methods.

Discomfort

The contact method provided less discomfort for the patient and in this respect proved superior to the noncontact method. The overdistension of the bowel with the danger of an ileus in highly stenotic tumors of the large bowel is virtually eliminated with the contact method. Pain, smoke, and laser-induced edema, often observed with the noncontact method and usually aggravating dysphagia for the first 24 hours, was either absent or much reduced with the contact method.

Damage to Material

With a certain measure of experience with the noncontact method, the danger of light guide combustion due to contamination of the tip is small, although the need to clean the tip occasionally during treatment prolongs the treatment session and wastes time.

We observed no ignition of fracture of the SLT sapphire tips in any patients treated by the contact method, although the tip regularly adhered to the irradiated tissue. The provision of continuous water irrigation improved matters (see Fig. **2**). We recommend, for the noncontact method, the use of white protective tips at the distal end of the endoscope (5). For the contact method, such protection of the distal end of the endoscope is not required (Table **1**).

Treatment Technique

The noncontact method has the advantage of permitting paintbrush, and not merely punctiform, irradiation by the laser. This is particularly important for large tumor masses and for exophytic tumor growth. In addition, the ability to work under visual control with the noncontact method represents significant advantage for laser therapy.

Table **1** Advantages and Disadvantages of the Contact and Noncontact Methods in the Clinical Practice of Nd:YAG Laser Therapy

	Contact	Versus	Noncontact	
+	no	Distension of the bowel	yes	−
+	no	Pain	yes	−
+	less	"Laser edema"	more	−
+	less	Smoke	more	−
+	no	Light guide ignition	yes	−
−	yes	Light guide adhesion	no	+
−	punctiform	Technique	"paint brush" application	+
−		Large tumour mass		+
−		Exophytic tumor		+
−	no	Therapy under direct vision	yes	+
−	yes	Tissue contact necessary	no	+
−		Tumor destruction from distal to proximal		+
+		from proximal to distal (with laser-resistant guide probe)		−
+		Total stenosis		−
+		Tumour overgrowth of the tube		−

The prerequisite for effective contact therapy is that the contact tip remains in uninterrupted contact with the tissue to be treated. Sometimes, this requirement can be only incompletely fulfilled, for example, in lesions associated with sharp angulations at the gastroesophageal junction. It also proved difficult to achieve proper tissue contact in the treatment of esophageal lesions, when the work was disturbed by respiratory excursions or aortic pulsations. In such cases it is usually easier to use the noncontact method, although the laser effect gained locally is more difficult to estimate owing to changes in the distance between the tip of the light guide and the tumor surface. However, this point does not seem particularly important in clinical practice, especially since the applied energy cannot always be reliably estimated even with the contact method when the sapphire tip is, for example, tangential to the tumor.

If the tumor stenosis could be negotiated endoscopically, the noncontact method proved superior to the contact method. Slow withdrawal of the endoscope allows irradiation of the tissue by the paintbrush technique, in a circular fashion and under direct vision, thus treating large tumor segments uniformly, without applying too much energy to any single site.

In total obstruction we prefer the contact method, since the sapphire tip can be advanced through the stenosis, opening up a narrow channel as it goes.

Important indications for the contact laser therapy are: highly stenotic benign or malignant lesions in the lower gastrointestinal tract with the possibility of avoiding coaxial gas insufflation with all the associated discomfort.

Finally, a relatively rare, but important, indication for the contact method is tumor overgrowth of endoprostheses. At laser power output of 80 W and more, as in the noncontact method, a short period of irradiation is enough to ignite the prosthesis and lead to toxic combustion fumes. With the contact method and its output of 10 to 20 W, this danger is avoided (Table **1**).

References

1. Daikuzono N, Joffe S: Artificial sapphire probe for contact photocoagulation and tissue vaporization with the Nd:YAG laser. Med Instrum 19 173–178, 1985

2. Delvaux M, Escourrou J: Complications observées au cours du traitement par laser des tumeurs du tractus digestif superieur. Acta Endosc 15:13, 1983

3. Ell C, Hochberger J, Lux G: Clinical experience of noncontact and contact Nd:YAG laser therapy for inoperable malignant stenoses of the oesophagus and stomach. Lasers Med Sci 1:143, 1986

4. Gourgouliatos Z, Wilcox B, Tores J, Motameli M, Rastegar S, Schwisinger W, Tio F, Welch AJ: Application of new laser probes in the treatment of gastrointestinal bleeding. (Abstr. 106.) Seventh Congress of the International Society for Laser Surgery and Medicine, Munich, 1987

5. Hochberger J, Ell C, Lux G: Protective tips for endoscopes used in laser therapy. Endoscopy 18:169, 1986

6. Naveau S, Zourabichvili O, Poynard T, Chaput JC: Comparison of an housed wave guide and naked wave guide for endoscopic Nd:YAG laser therapy for esophageal and rectal tumorus: A randomized clinical trial. (Abstr. 51.) Third Congress of European Laser Association, Amsterdam, November 6–8, 1986

7. Sabben G, Lambert R, Lenz P: Lasertherapy with fibres in tissue contact. Gastrointest Endosc 29:183, 1983

8. Steger AC, Moore KC, Hiva N: The place of the low power contact Nd:YAG technique in the treatment of inoperable oesophageal and rectal cancers. (Abstr. 111c.) Seventh Congress of the International Society for Laser Surgery and Medicine, Munich 1987

9. Suzuki S, Aoki J, Shiina Y, Nomiyama T, Miwa T: New ceramic endoprobes for endoscopic contact irradiation with Nd:YAG laser: Experimental studies and clinical application. Gastrointest Endosc 32:282, 1986

10. Tsujimura D, Kagen H, Matsui H, Hajiro K, Yamamoto T, Daikuzono N: Contact methods or endoscopic laser treatment. Proceedings of 7th international Congress "Laser 85, Opto-Electronic," Munich, July, 1985 (p 352)

11. Tsunekawa H, Morise K, Iizuka A, et al: Studies on the application of the newly developed laser microprobes for the Nd:YAG laser endoscopy. Proceedings of 7th International Congress "Laser 85, Opto-Electronik," Munich, July, 1985

Interstitial Laser Therapy

S. G. Bown

Lasers are high-technology instruments that can deliver light energy to tissue with a great deal of precision. However, many of their current clinical applications, although more accurate than the available alternatives, are still relatively crude. In current endoscopic practice in gastroenterology, lasers are used essentially like surgical instruments, the effects being judged largely just on the immediate visual changes. The real future of lasers in medicine lies in harnessing the precision available and applying it to biologic systems. Inevitably, it is far more difficult to control all the factors that influence the nature and extent of laser effects in living tissue than it is in inanimate materials, but one can do considerably better than with other energy sources, such as diathermy. Major advances over current clinical practice can be made by reducing the neodymium:yttrium-aluminum-garnet (Nd:YAG) laser power from 50 to 80 W used to palliate advanced, obstructing tumors to just 1 to 2 W, and using a bare fiber delivery system whose tip can be inserted directly into tissue. This is known as interstitial hyperthermia, and its use with the Nd:YAG laser was first reported in 1983 (1).

Predictability of Biologic Effects

The energy delivered to tissue from a laser is easy to control. The distribution of energy within the target depends on the optical properties of the tissue, which determine how the light is reflected, transmitted, scattered, or absorbed. In early experiments to assess the high power Nd:YAG laser for control of gastrointestinal hemorrhage, it was shown that the depth of damage to the stomach wall depended closely on the total energy applied (2, 8), whereas with diathermy techniques there was much more variation; although, in general, more diathermy energy causes more damage, low energies could cause full-thickness damage, whereas in other lesions high energies did not necessarily produce any changes in the external muscle layer (15). The range of biologic responses to local heat from a high-power laser with a deeply penetrating wavelength, like the infrared beam of the Nd:YAG laser at 1064 nm, can be summarized as:

Total destruction: Instant vaporization
                             Necrosis with later
                             sloughing
Destruction with   Necrosis with healing by
reconstruction: scarring
                             Necrosis with healing by
                             regeneration
Reversible effects: Edema and inflammation
                             Local warming only

Under appropriate circumstances, all these effects can be seen in the same organ. For example, a Nd:YAG shot of 3 s at 70 W onto a 3 mm spot on normal stomach wall will instantly vaporize a small area of mucosa, necrose the muscularis mucosae and submucosa, which slough over a few days, and cause partial necrosis in the external muscle layer, which heals with fibrosis, whereas there is regeneration of the mucosa and submucosa. This same range of effects can be seen in neoplastic tissue (1). This has major therapeutic implications, since it means that there is the potential for destroying localized tumors, particularly in thin-walled organs, and replacing the diseased tissue either with a scar or by regeneration of the normal tissue. For this to be a practical proposition, one must be sure that one is indeed going to leave a scar rather than finish up with a perforation, and the experimental data so far available to answer this question are limited. The extent of lesions produced with particular laser parameters is reasonably predictable with the high-power laser. However, with the low-power laser, no vaporization is seen, and there is much gentler and more prolonged tissue hyperthermia that is easier to control and gives much greater precision.

Interstitial Laser Therapy

The concept of interstitial therapy opens a whole new range of lesions to the possibility of laser treatment. The idea is very simple. Instead of delivering light from a noncontact fiber or by a tip in contact with the tissue surface, the fiber is inserted directly into the target organ. By this means, the maximum response can be centered anywhere within the organ and there need be little effect actually at the surface apart from the small hole required for fiber insertion. This can be extremely valuable, although it does mean that it is impossible to assess the results of treatment by the immediate visual effect. For this to be safe, it is essential to be able to predict the nature, extent, and healing of the tissue damage that given treatment parameters will produce. This approach is likely to be most suitable for tumors of solid organs such as the liver and prancreas, although it might also be useful for more solid lesions in the walls of hollow organs, such as sessile villous adenomas in the colon.

When the fiber tip is buried in tissue, the response occurs in a very confined space. If the energy is delivered too fast, the result can be drastic, for if any water is vaporized, there is nowhere for it to escape, which can lead to local pressure disruption. Also, the tip can be damaged if it gets too hot while in contact with biologic material. Thus, interstitial therapy is best carried out at very low laser powers (less than 5 W).

Liver

Little work has yet been done on interstitial hyperthermia with lasers in any organ, but the best documented experimental data so far available are those of Matthewson et al (12) in studies of the rat liver. They chose a simple experimental model in which a 0.4 mm diameter fiber from a low-power Nd:YAG laser was inserted directly into the center of a lobe of liver, exposed at laparotomy, in Wistar rats. They originally used a pulsed laser (0.1 ms pulses at 40 Hz), but subsequently showed that the results were identical to those with a continuous wave laser (11). Lesions were made in the liver using a range of laser powers and exposure times, and the animals were killed at varying times after treatment to assess how the size of the necrotic area produced depended on the laser parameters used and how these lesions healed. Further experiments used an array of microthermocouples to measure the temperature distribution up to 8 mm from the fiber tip during laser exposure. The results of these experiments can be summarized as follows:

Well-defined areas of necrosis, roughly spherical in shape and up to 16 mm in diameter, could be produced around each treatment point.

The diameter of each zone of necrosis was predictable and depended on the laser power and exposure time used.

At powers more than 1 W, charring occurred around the fiber tip.

All lesions healed by regeneration, without complication, within 60 days, leaving a small scar.

The steady-state temperature during laser exposure at the edge of the final zone of necrosis varied with the exposure time and was the same as that found with other ways of applying hypertheremia (e.g., for a 30-minute exposure, the termperature at the edge of the zone of necrosis was 44°C).

The volume of necrosis from each treatment site is small, and it remains to be seen whether this can be enlarged by using more sophisticated fiber tips, such as sapphires or diffuser tips (5). This work was limited to normal liver in small animals. Similar lesions can be produced in malignant tissue (9), and it is likely that necrosed tumor in the liver will heal in the same way as necrosed normal tissue, with regeneration of liver and some scarring, although this has not yet been demonstrated. A more difficult question is whether areas of necrosis in the liver of larger animals or man will heal as well as those in the rat. Also, no work has yet been done using multiple adjacent sites, treated simultaneously or consecutively, as would be required to treat lesions of the size likely to be attained by hepatic tumors in man. However, the concept of destroying intrahepatic tumors simply by inserting a series of laser fibers into the lesion to provide local hyperthermia is very exciting. It would seem most suitable for single lesions, either primary hepatomas or isolated metastases, the extent of the neoplasm within the mass of the liver being identified by ultrasound. Early treatments would be done at laparotomy, but it is conceivable that the technique could be developed for use at laparoscopy, or even with direct percutaneous access under ultrasound control, as is currently used to biopsy difficult intrahepatic lesions. So far, there has been only one preliminary clinical report, from Japan, in which ten primary or secondary intrahepatic tumors were treated interstitially with a low-power Nd:YAG laser at laparotomy (7). There were no serious complications and the two patients with primary hepatomas had a dramatic reduction in the serum levels of alpha-fetoprotein, indicating a major reduction in tumor bulk. If further work shows that this idea is effective and safe, it could represent a major advance because the current surgical alternatives, partial hepatectomy and transplantation, are considerably more complicated and hazardous, and chemotherapy is far from entirely satisfactory.

Pancreas

Pancreatic cancer has a poor prognosis. Very few are resectable, and few respond to chemotherapy or radiotherapy, so any new form of treatment that does not involve pancreatic resection could represent a significant advance. Surgical access (as opposed to resection) is relatively easy, so insertion of laser fibers for local hyperthermia would present no problem. The major unknown factor is how normal and neoplastic pancreatic tissue will respond to thermal necrosis. There is a very definite risk of fistula formation, hemorrhagic pancreatitis, and infection in necrotic areas leading to pancreatic abscesses. Nevertheless, preliminary experiments (14) show that local necrosis can be produced in the normal dog pancreas, which heals safely with fibrosis, but hemorrhagic pancreatitis does occur and it has not yet been established whether it is possible to avoid the pancreatitis in a predictable manner. This is an area of current active research.

Colon

Hollow organs like the colon do not lend themselves to interstitial therapy as readily as solid organs like the liver and pancreas. However, some solid tumors of the colon, such as sessile adenomas or sessile malignant polyps, are unsuitable for alternative endoscopic treatment and in patients unfit for surgery the gentle and precise necrosis offered by low-power hyperthermia may prove useful. Matthewson et al. (10) have assessed this in rats, comparing the tissue responses of normal colon and dimethyldhydrazine-induced colon carcinomas. Normal tissue was vulnerable, and with the laser fiber just touching the mucosa, 1 W for 75 or 100 s caused full-thickness necrosis and a significant reduction in the bursting pressure of the colon. These lesions healed over 3 weeks with a small amount of fibrosis. Necrosis in the tumors was produced by inserting the fiber about 2 mm into the tumor and using similar laser parameters (1 W for up to 400 s, depending on the size of the tumor). Measurement of the tumor size was difficult, since treatment was carried out endoscopically (using a pediatric bronchoscope), so determining the exposure time to give necrosis that matched the extent of the tumor being treated was not easy. Overtreatment caused colon perforation, undertreatment left residual tumor, but when the exposure time was correct, complete tumor necrosis occurred, leaving a shallow ulcer that healed completely in 4 weeks.

This is a new approach to laser treatment of gastrointestinal tract tumors and has not yet been assessed clinically, but could prove to be a useful advance. Only a low-power laser is required, and the treatment is less uncomfortable than conventional high-power laser techniques for patient and endoscopist, since there is no smoke production and no coaxial gas is required around the laser fiber. The development of sapphire tips for laser fibers (3) brought the laser power down from 50 to 80 W to 10 to 15 W, and put the fiber tip in contact with the tissue surface (13). Interstitial hyperthermia has gone one stage further, bringing the laser power down by a further factor of 10 and delivering the laser energy to the center rather than the surface of solid organs.

In theory, any solid tumor accessible to single or multiple laser fibers directly, surgically or endoscopically, is a candidate for interstitial therapy, but before it becomes a realistic proposal, one must be able to satisfy the basic criteria that the extent of the necrosis must match the extent of the lesion being treated and structure and function must be acceptable at all stages of healing.

Technological Developments

Most of the major developments in medicine and surgery over the last 40 years have come from the application of science and technology to clinical problems. However, to get the maximum value from this joining of forces between clinical and nonclinical expertise, the level of understanding of the effects involved must be comparable on each side of the fence. With regard to medical lasers, at present this is not the case. The instruments currently available give well-defined and precisely controllable light outputs, whereas the clinical effects are often judged on a purely empirical basis. Some laser applications, particularly in specialities such as ophthalmology, are carried out with a high degree of sophistication, but most of the current endoscopic work on recanalizing advanced obstructing tumors of the gastrointestinal tract is relatively crude. It is safe and effective and is appropriate for the patients being treated, but it is not making maximum use of the precision available from the instruments. To redress this balance, the urgent need is for experiments to obtain much better quantification of immediate and delayed effects of laser light on living tissue. These are likely to prove most rewarding for low-power hyperthermia, as described in this chapter, and for photodynamic therapy, as described elsewhere in this book.

Even if technology is currently ahead of the clinicians, there is still plenty of work for the physicists and engineers to do. There is plenty of scope for improving the efficiency and reliability of current lasers and increasing the range of fiberoptic delivery systems to match the rapidly expanding range of applications. Probably the three most important areas in the short term are stable, low-power lasers, fiber tips, and multifiber systems. However, looking further into the future, the greatest technologic challenge will be the development of feedback and control systems. A simple example of this would be with sapphire fiber tips. These get hot during use, and the actual temperature will depend on the laser power, duration of application, tip cooling system (gas or water), and what material is in contact with the tip. If the sapphire is not hot enough, it will not produce the desired cutting effect, and if it is too hot, tissue will stick to it and impede surgery. Probably, the ideal temperature is about 80°C. However, the biologic material touching the tip is continuously changing, either because the tip is moving or because the tissue is changing under the influence of the applied light beam. This problem could be solved by having a microthermocouple built into the sapphire to monitor its temperature continuously, and designing a feedback system that would adjust the laser power to maintain the sapphire at the optimum temperature.

More sophisticated systems would be required to monitor temperatures and light fluences within tissue. Tissue necrosis from hyperthermia depends on both the temperature reached and on the time that that temperature is maintained. As an approximation, hyperthermia kills exponentially as a function of time at temperatures higher than 42°C. Increasing the temperature by 1°C halves the time required to kill cells (6). Experimental data are not yet available to say whether the same is true for tumors, but it seems likely that it would be, particularly for the areas of tumor most important for treatment if there is to be any prospect of complete eradication, namely, the regions where the tumor is invading adjacent normal tissue. Thus, one can envisage computer-controlled ablation of tumors in such organs as the liver and pancreas. Local hyperthermia is provided by an array of interstitial laser fibers distributed through the tumor so that all neoplastic areas are sufficiently close to a fiber (probably within about 1 cm) for high enough therapeutic temperatures to be reached. The extent of tumor invasion is established by intraoperative ultrasound (or by earlier computed tomography or nuclear magnetic resonance scans) and a separate array of thermocouples are placed at strategic points on the tumor margin to monitor tissue temperature. The computer integrates the temperature and the time during which that temperature is maintained for each thermocouple, and when the total exceeds that required to produce necrosis at each thermocouple, the laser power is turned off. This approach to cancer treatment may sound very futuristic, but there is no fundamental reason why it should not be achievable in the relatively near future and a prototype system has already been reported (4). The simpler approach of using a multifiber system but without feedback control could become practical even sooner, although it would require longer treatment times to ensure adequate necrosis, particularly at the tumor margin. Nevertheless, one must always remember that concepts of treatment like this are only attainable if the biologic data are available for the normal and neoplastic tissues involved to say what combination of temperature and treatment time causes the tissue necrosis that is required for safe healing.

References

1. Bown SG: Phototherapy of tumours. World J Surg 7:700–707, 1983
2. Bown SG, Salmon PR, Storey DW, et al: NdYAG laser photocoagulation in the dog stomach. GUT 21:818–825, 1980
3. Daikozono N, Joffe SN: An artificial sapphire probe for contact photocoagulation and tissue vaporisation using the NdYAG laser. Med Instrum 19:173–178, 1985
4. Daikozono N, Joffe SN: Computer controlled contact NdYAG laser system for interstitial local hyperthermia. Lasers Med Surg 6:216, 1986
5. Fujii H, Asakura T, Jutamulia S, Kaneko S, Tsuru M: Light scattering properties of a roughened optical fibre. Opt Laser Technol 16:40, 1984
6. Hahn GM: Hyperthermia and Cancer. Plenum Press, New York 1982
7. Hashimoto D, Takami M, Idezuki Y: In depth radiation therapy by YAG laser for malignant tumours in the liver under ultrasound imaging. Gastroenterology 88:1663, 1985
8. Kelly DF, Bown SG, Calder BM, Pearson H, Weaver BMQ, Swain CP, Salmon PR: Histological changes following NdYAG laser photocoagulation of canine gastric mucosa. GUT 24:914–920, 1983
9. Matthewson K, Barr H, Tralau CJ, Bown SG: Interstitial low powered NdYAG laser therapy studies in a transplanted rat fibrosarcoma. Br J Surg (in press)
10. Matthewson K, Barton T, Lewin MR, O'Sullivan JP, Northfield TC, Bown SG: Low power interstitial NdYAG laser photocoagulation in normal and neoplastic rat colon. GUT 29:27–34, 1988
11. Matthewson K, Coleridge-Smith P, Northfield TC, Bown SG: Comparison of continuous wave and pulsed excitation for interstitial NdYAG laser induced hyperthermia. Lasers Med Sci 1:197–201, 1986
12. Matthewson K, Coleridge-Smith PD, O'Sullivan JP, Northfield TC, Bown SG: Biological effects of intrahepatic NdYAG laser photocoagulation in rats. Gastroenterology 93: 550–557, 1987
13. Rutgeerts P, Vantrappen G, D'Heygere F, Geboes K: Endoscopic contact NdYAG laser therapy for colorectal cancer – a randomised comparison with non-contact therapy. Lasers Med Sci 2: 69–72, 1987
14. Steger A, Barr H, Hawes R et al: Experimental studies on interstitial hyperthermia for treating pancreatic cancer. GUT 28: 1382, 1987
15. Swain CP, Mills TN, Shemesh E, et al: Which electrode? A comparison of four endoscopic methods of electrocoagulation in experimental bleeding ulcers. GUT 25:1424–1431, 1984

Ultrasonographically Guided Lasers and Spheric Lasers

D. Hashimoto

Neodymium:yttrium-aluminum-garnet (Nd: YAG) laser has been used for the treatment of tumors on hollow organs through endoscopy, whereas, due to its property of rectilinear propagation, it has not been thought suitable for the treamtent of tumors in parenchymatous tissue.

Based on the premise that if Nd:YAG laser could be radiated spherically, one could produce a round coagulation of tissue that could be visualized by ultrasonic imaging, we developed a new method of laser therapy for liver cancers using in-depth spherical radiation (1, 2).

Shape of the Fiber Tip

In order to obtain the optimum fiber tip for spherically dispersed radiation, computer simulated ray tracing was performed. The data from simulated optical ray tracing performed on 20000 rays with varying conical angles showed that a single conical tip did not produce uniform spherical radiation.

Therefore, computer simulation was used to assess a double conical tip. In order to further improve the uniformity of radiation, we introduced new parameters, the first conical angle, theta 1, the second conical angle, theta 2, and the tip radius, R, into the computer ray trace software. Based on the simulation results, probes with theta 1 = 70, theta 2 = 30, and R = 0.3 mm were manufactured (Fig. 1).

Judging from the actual radiation pattern of this probe, the computer simulated results seemed to be satisfactory.

Optimal Conditions for Radiation

Analyses of the relationship between laser power and coagulated shape showed that as the laser power increases, the shape of the tissue coagulated becomes more oval, whereas, as the laser power decreases, the tissue coagulated becomes more round.

After much experimentation, approximately 5 W continuous radiation energy proved to be optimal (Fig. 2).

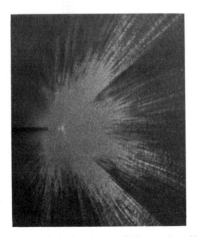
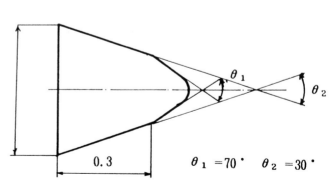

θ_1 θ_2

0.3 $\theta_1 = 70°$ $\theta_2 = 30°$

Fig. **1**   Spherical laser radiation probe with double conical tapered tip and round end.

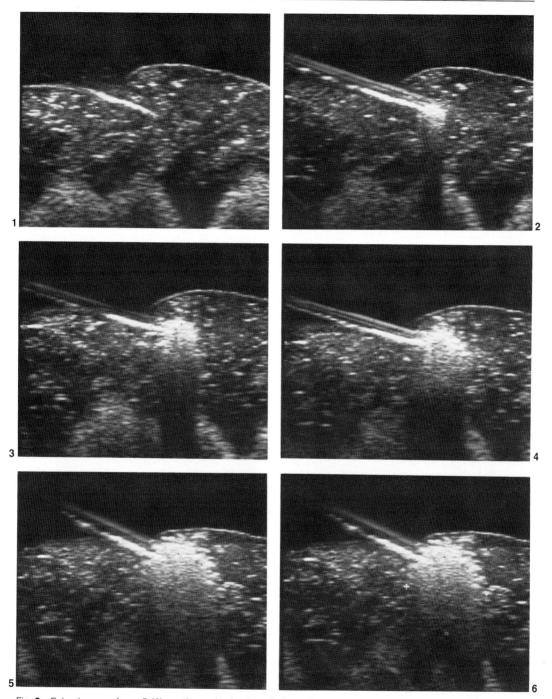

Fig. 2 Echo images from 5 W continous in-depth radiation of resected bovine liver at 1, 3, 5, 10, 20, and 30 minutes.

With 5 W continuous laser radiation, approximately 500 J/cm³ proved to be adequate to coagulate a circle of tissue in the case of canine resected liver. In living canine liver, 1000 J/cm³ was necessary to coagulate the same size of tissue. Due to the cooling effect of blood flow, different laser energies seemed to be required for achieving the same amount of coagulated round tissue.

Gas Formation

During in-depth spherical radiation, the temperature around the tip of the fiber probe reaches 200° to 300°C, and mixed gases including carbon dioxide, water, melcapthane, methylamine, and aldehyde were generated. During tissue vaporization, hot and high-pressure vapor may cause gas embolism in intrahepatic vessels or heat burn of intrahepatic bile ducts.

To resolve these serious problems, a gas evacuation device was made in the form of a T-shaped tube. The T-tube was connected to a pump to apply negative pressure. By applying 10 cm Hg negative pressure, gas generated around the fiber tip was completely removed.

Histologic Changes

Histologic changes of coagulated tissue were analyzed on normal canine liver.

After in-depth spherical radiation, a black carbonized layer with a cavity in its center and thick, white coagulated layers surrounding it were observed. Histologically, hepatocytes were completely necrotized in the coagulated tissue, and the boundary between coagulated tissue and normal liver tissue surrounding it was clearly observed. In 1 week, thin fibrous tissue with prominent inflammatory cell infiltration formed on the boundary. Central to this, massive hepatocyte necrosis with vacuolation and denucleation were observed microscopically. In 1 month, the fibrous tissue thickened, and pseudo-bile ducts proliferated at the periphery of the fibrous tissue. Neither bleeding, bile leakage, nor abscess formation were observed.

In-Depth Temperature Measurement

We have developed an in-depth temperature measurement device to analyze the thermal distribution of radiated tissue. The device con-

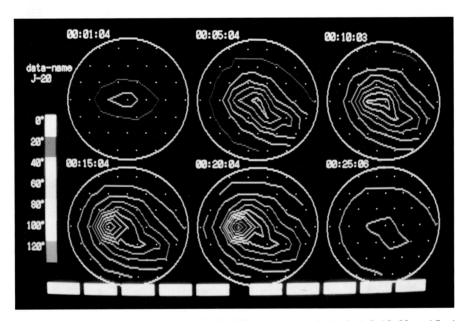

Fig. 3 Temperature measurements during in-depth 5 W continuous radiation in 1, 5, 10, 20, and 5 minutes after laser switch off.

sists of 37 thermocouples, which were equally spaced 7 mm apart. The temperatures measured by these thermocouples were processed by a computer through a data-logger interface and displayed on a CRT monitor. When continuous radiation was applied at 5 W, the expansion of isothermal lines was observed to coincide with enlargement of the highly echoic area (Fig. **3**).

According to the in-depth measured data, the temperature of the probe tip was 240° to 360 °C. That of the white coagulated tissue was approximately 50° to 60 °C, and that of the carbonized layers was in the range of 100° to 160°.

Ultrasonic Observation

The importance of ultrasonic imaging in laser therapy is:

– Guidance of liver puncture
– Decision of energy required
– Assessment of coagulated area
– Monitoring of gas formation

Liver puncture can be performed under ultrasonic guidance. For puncturing, we applied a 15 gauge Teflon needle 30 cm in length. In order to improve echogenicity, surface roughness of the Teflon canula was increased. Before deciding on the puncturing direction, prepuncture in water was performed to set up the guideline on the monitor of the ultrasonic imaging system. The tumor to be irradiated can be aimed at accurately by aligning it on the guideline preset on the monitor.

Assuming the tumor to be a sphere, the maximum diameter can be determined by echo image, and the approximate maximum volume of the tumor can be calculated. The amount of energy to be applied can be determined assuming 1000 J/cm³. The time necessary for treatment can be determined by dividing the required energy by 5 W.

The assessment of coagulated area should be carried out via echoic images made of various sections, especially in cases in which a tumor has an irregular shape.

During radiation, when gas is not continuously evacuated, microbubbles are observed around the tissue coagulated. In such cases, radiation should be stopped to recheck the evacuation system.

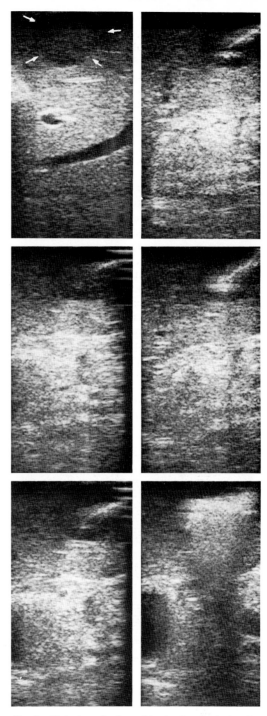

Fig. **4** Clinical application of in-depth spherical radiation on metastatic liver cancer originated from gastric cancer.

Clinical Application

Six cases of hepatocellular carcinoma were successfully treated at laparotomy. In cases in which more than $1000\,J/cm^3$ per unit tumor volume were successfully applied, alpha-feto-protein decreased dramatically and reached normal range.

In-depth spherical laser therapy at laparotomy has the following advantages: Intraoperative ultrasonography can detect new small liver cancers that were not detectable by preoperative extracorporeal ultrasound; and in-depth spherical laser radiation therapy is more effective and safer because respiratory excursions are automatically followed by the laser, and as a result the laser does not move in relation to the target tissue.

In-depht spherical laser radiation therapy was applied in eigth cases of metastatic liver cancer in order to decrease tumor volume (Fig. **4**). In these cases, because of multiplicity of cancer and limitations of tumor detectability of small cancers less than 1 cm by ultrasound, selective chemotherapy or selective immunotherapy were applied additionally.

Future Trends

With rapid progress being made in imaging technologies, such as ultrasonics, computed tomography, nuclear magnetic resonance, digital substraction angiography, detection of early liver cancers has become much easier. However, it is still difficult to assess cancers decisively in their early stage with one single imaging modality because of the varied types of cancer tissue. Not only ultrasonographic guidance but various imaging techniques should take an important part in the in-depth spherical laser radiation therapy.

In-depth spherical laser radiation therapy has the following advantages:

- Selective treatment of cancer with no bleeding and no bile leakage
- Availability for laparoscopic or percutaneous transhepatic approach, depending on the patient's operability
- Local curability of a cancer with less than 5 mm diameter without any shift of the fiber tip

The future trend in development will be an establishment of the automatic puncture techniques to prevent unfavorable damages of the intrahepatic vessels and the bile ducts. Various types of medical images such as the MRI and the stereoscopic angiographs could be graphically multiplied to give a three-dimentional scope of the operational area. Being input the intraoperative medical images and resembled with preoperatively input data during the operation, the puncture of the laser probe will be carried out percutaneously with much safer and easier manner.

References

1. Hashimoto D, Takami M, Idezuki Y: In-depth radiation therapy by YAG laser for malignant tumors in the liver under ultrasonic imaging. Proceedings of 4th meeting of the World Federation for Ultrasound in Medicine and Biology 1985 (p 78)
2. Hashimoto D, Yabe K, Uedera U, Idezuki Y: New laser puncture therapy for liver cancers. Nd:YAG Laser in Medicine and Surgery

Laser-Resistant Guide Probe

J. Hochberger, J. F. Riemann, and C. Ell

The foreword application laser energy in highly stenotic tumors, as recommended in the initial stages of laser therapy in the gastrointestinal tract (5–7), may carry a significant risk of a "via falsa". Exophytically growing tumor tissue, natural bends in the areas of the esophagus and stomach or colon, and edema development during laser therapy make the evaluation of the position of the natural lumen of a narrowed section of the intestine more difficult. The incidence of complications of 15 to 30% may be partly explained by this fact (1, 7, 10).

With the aim of making palliative endoscopic laser therapy of non-passable marked stenoses safer and also more comfortable for the patient, we developed a laser-resistant probe that serves simultaneously as guide for orientation during laser irradiation and as an aspiration and irrigation device (3, 9).

Probe Material and Construction

When looking for suitable laser-resistant probe material, it has to be kept in mind that in endoscopic application of the neodymium:yttrium-aluminum-garnet (Nd:YAG) laser with the non-contact method, temperatures of more than 1000°C will be reached in the vaporization of tissue by laser (8, 9). Therefore, the material to be used for the probe has to be resistant to direct laser irradiation as well as the high temperatures induced by the vaporization of tissue surrounding the probe. Furthermore, the material used must have a low heat conductivity in order to prevent thermal damage to the healthy tissue and to the endoscope.

Altogether, the probe material must meet the following requirements: low absorption of laser light of a wavelength of 1064 nm, high resistance to heat, low heat conductivity, sufficient mechanical stability (in a probe diameter of less than 2.6 mm), and biocompatibility. In comprehensive tests of different materials, various precious metals, metal alloys of low heart conductivity, plastics, glass and quartz, glass ceramics, and bioceramic materials were tested (9). Aluminium oxide (Al_2O_3) bioceramics proved to be advantageous as basic substance. The material, which appears white to the eye, is very hard and corresponds approximately to polycrystaline sapphire in its chemical compostion and its physical properties. Aluminium oxide has a melting point of 2043°C, is applied in many fields as insulating material because of its low thermal conductivity and is used as biomedical implant material in various surgical disciplines. Even in the small dimensions necessary for use in endoscopes, a good mechanical strength of the material has been shown. The laser-resistant guide probe is mainly divided into three different sections: The laser-resistant part of the probe (10 cm), the highly flexible probe tip, and the end part of the probe of about 1.8 m in length (Fig. 1).

In order to achieve a sufficiently high flexibility in the laser-resistant section of the probe, cylindroid ceramic pearls of about 4 mm in length with a central longitudinal drill hole were manufactured. These pearls were then strung on a highly temperature-resistant and highly reflecting metal wire on a tungsten or platinum basis (melting points: tungsten [pure metal] 3380°C, platinum [pure metal] 1769°C). The pearls are kept together by a spring tension mechanism. In order to allow the correct placing of the probe without risking perforation even in marked stenoses with very irregular lumina, the distal end of the probe was given a highly flexible and soft guide wire approximately 10 cm long with a diameter of 0.9 mm. In the proximal section, the laser-resistant part of the probe is first connected with an aspiration tube that is, in turn, con-

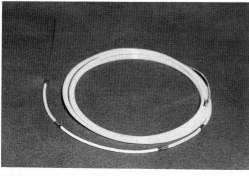

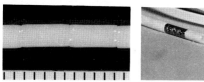

Fig. **1** Laser-resistant probe with highly flexible probe tip (left), laser-resistant probe section consisting of bioceramic pearls (center), aspiration tube with endpart of a hollow catheter (right).

nected to a Teflon hollow catheter of 1.8 m in length. Through this catheter, insufflated gas, smoke, or liquid can be removed or, alternatively, contrast media or liquid can be instilled.

Clinical Application

In practice, the following procedure proved useful for the application in a standard endoscope with a single instrumentation channel (Fig. **2**). The probe is passed via the instrumentation channel and then placed under direct vision and possibly under additional radiologic control through the endoscopically non-passable tumor stenosis so that the laser-resistant ceramic part lies in the area of the stenosis to be irradiated. The endoscope is then removed with the probe remaining in position and is then, in a second procedure, reintroduced next to the probe up to the site of the tumor stenosis. The light guide is then passed via the free instrumentation channel and the stenosis is irradiated tangentially to the guide probe, circling it until the stenosis can be passed with the endoscope or until the poststenotic lumen can be seen.

When a two-channel endoscope is used, the two insertions of the endoscope are not necessary. However, we found this procedure not advisable because of the larger caliber of these endoscopes. For safety reasons, especially in direct irradiation of the laser probe, a laser output of not more than 70 W in the noncontact method is to be recommended for irradiation alongside the laser-resistant guide. Also for safety reasons, the probe is as a rule only used once. When contact tips are used, such safety recommendations are not necessary.

To date, this laser-resistant guide probe was used in 16 patients in 34 sessions without any complications. Ten patients underwent laser therapy in the lower gastrointestinal tract

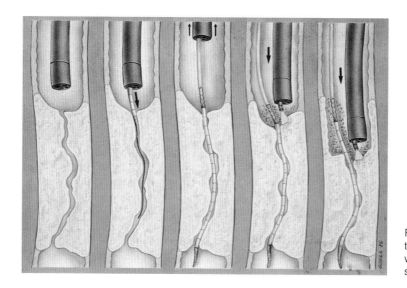

Fig. **2** Placing and use of the laser-resistant probe with a single-channel endoscope.

and six patients in the upper tract. The following clinical example illustrates the usefulness of the laser-resistant guide in defined situations. A 47-year-old patient with leiomyosarcoma of the small intestine and infiltration of the large bowel was admitted to the hospital because of a marked narrowing in the area of the sigmoid. It was not possible to dilate the stenosis of only 3 to 4 mm in diameter with a bougienage-coloscope. The mechanical irritation involved in the attempt to open the stenosis with the endoscope caused a mucosal swelling that almost completely closed it (Fig. 3). Because of air insufflation during colonoscopy, a very painful overdistension of the entire colon developed (Fig. 4). Therefore, as a first measure, the laser-resistant guide probe was placed through the stenosis under endoscopic vision and the insufflated air was aspirated. The patient was immediately free of pain (Fig. 5). Then laser therapy using the contact method alongside the laser-resistant

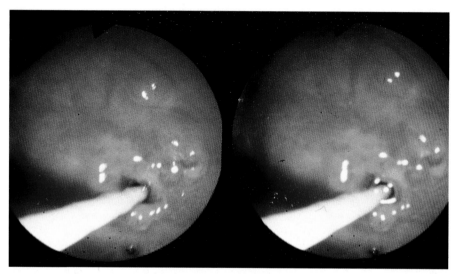

Fig. 3   Marked sigmoid stenosis (width of lumen, 3 mm), laser-resistant guide probe in situ.

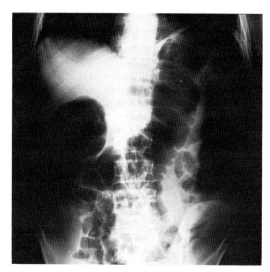

Fig. 4   Massive distension of the whole large bowel proximal to the stenosis.

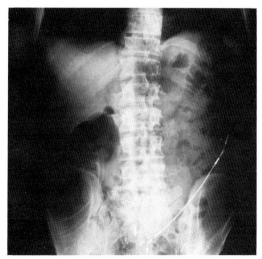

Fig. 5   Aspiration via the laser-resistant guide probe.

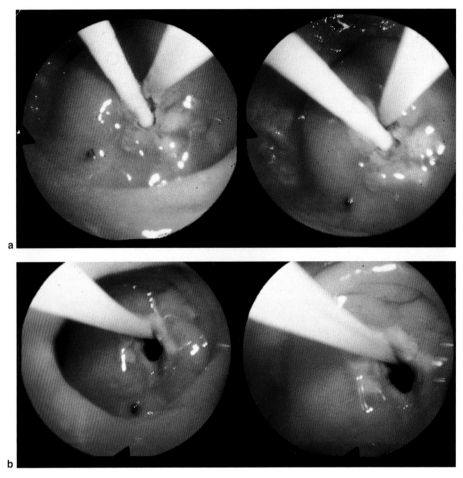

a

b

Fig. **6a, b**   Laser therapy along the laser guide with the contact method (with liquid irrigation of the light guide).

probe was started with water as light guide irrigation medium (Figs. **6**). The insufflated air was removed intermittently during this treatment by passing the laser-resistant probe into the proximal part of the intestine. After two laser sessions, the stenosis could then be passed with a small-calibre endoscope (Olympus PCF).

Discussion

The question of using a guide probe in laser therapy of highly stenotic tumors that cannot be passed endoscopically may arise, but it is difficult to find suitable material for the probe. The use of a probe made of metal, as suggested by Wood and Innes (11) is dangerous,

since heat conduction along the probe can lead to extended burning or damage to the intestine close to the probe or the endoscope. In comprehensive material studies, bioceramics proved to be a suitable substance, meeting the material requirements sufficiently. It has low thermal conductivity, low absorption of laser light of a wavelength of 1064 nm, tolerates high temperatures, with a melting point greater than 2000 °C, and is biocompatible.

In marked, endoscopically nonpassable stenoses of the upper gastrointestinal tract the combination of bougienage following retrograde laser therapy under lumen vision has contributed to reducing the risk and, now, is generally accepted (2, 4). As our experiences show, even if they are only limited in number, it seems possible to shorten the treatment procedure (no bougienage, fewer laser sessions) by using the laser probe without increasing the risk of perforation for the patient. A comparative prospective study of the two treatment techniques is however necessary before the laser guide probe can be generally recommended for highly stenotic tumors in the upper gastrointestinal tract.

At the moment, the laser-resistant probe is, without doubt, favored for the use in marked, endoscopically nonpassable stenoses in the lower gastrointestinal tract, since bougienage is usually not a possible alternative there. Furthermore, this area shows more natural bends compared with the upper gastrointestinal tract, especially in the area of the rectosigmoid. As a rule, the integrated aspiration and irrigation device relieves the physician of the dangerous obligation to open the stenosis in one single session: the prestenotic, usually extremely painful distension of the bowel or the danger of an ileus can be avoided by intermittent aspiration combined with irrigation if necessary.

References

1. Delvaux M, Escourrou J: Complications observées au cours du traitement par laser des tumeurs du tractus digestif superieur. Acta Endosc 15: 13, 1985

2. Ell C, Demling L: Laser therapy in the upper GI-tract. Laser Surg Med 7: 491–494, 1987

3. Ell C, Hochberger J, Riemann JF, Lux G, Demling L: Laser-resistant guide probe for laser treatment of endoscopically impassable tumour stenoses. Endoscopy 18: 27, 1986

4. Ell C, Riemann G, Lux L, Demling L: Palliative laser treatment of malignant stenoses in the upper gastrointestinal tract. Endoscopy 28 (Suppl 1): 21, 1986

5. Fleischer D: Endoscopic Nd:YAG laser therapy for diseases of the esophagus. In: Joffe SN, Mukkerheide J, Goldman L (eds): Neodymium YAG Laser in Medicine and Surgery. Elsevier, Amsterdam 1983 (p 42)

6. Fleischer D, Kessler F: Endoscopic Nd:YAG laser therapy for carcinoma of the esophagus: A new form of palliative treatment. Gastroenterology 85: 600, 1983

7. Fleischer D, Sivak M: Endoscopic Nd:YAG laser palliation for obstructing esophagogastric carcinoma. Lasers Surg Med 3: 172, 1983

8. Goosens A, Enderby C: Fundamentals of medical lasers. Gastrointest Endosc 30: 74, 1984

9. Hochberger J: Entwicklung, Konstruktion und erster klinischer Einsatz einer laserfesten Führungssonde zur Verbesserung der Therapie von Stenosen des Gastrointestinaltraktes mit dem Neodym-YAG-Laser. Inaugural Disseration, University of Erlangen-Nuernberg, 1987

10. Mosquet L, Brunetaud JM: Les lasers en gastroentérologie: faut-il s'équiper et lequel choisir? Gastroenterol Clin Biol 8: 138, 1984

11. Wood JW, Innes JW: Tumor ablation by endoscopic Nd:YAG laser. Am J Gastroenterol 80: 715, 1985

The 1.32 μm Nd:YAG Laser: A New Laser in Gastroenterology

J. Hochberger and C. Ell

All neodymium:yttrium-aluminum-garnet (Nd:YAG) laser systems used so far in gastroenterology work at a wavelength of 1.064 μm. It is possible, though, to change a standard Nd:YAG laser to emit light of a wavelength of 1.32 μm by modifying the resonator. Habitually in the Nd:YAG laser, as a four-level laser system, only the most effective atomic transition with a light emission at 1.064 μm is used, and the creation of other different wavelengths is suppressed. A transition of the neodymium ions from the excited pump band state to the ground state emitting a different light can be attained by using highly selective dielectric mirrors or dispersion prisms in the resonator. In this way it is possible to create light oscillations at 1.32 μm. However, even in a high-efficiency continuous wave laser system, the energy output will only be about 25% (3).

The starting point for tests with a laser of a wavelength of 1.32 μm is the changed optical properties of tissue at this wavelength in comparison to the wavelength of 1.064 μm, and the resulting different tissue effects. Whereas at 1.32 μm wavelength the light extinction, i.e., the weakening by absorption and diffusion in blood, is reduced by the factor 3 in blood compared with 1.064 μm, the energy absorption in water is increased by the factor 10 (8). Against this physical background, a change of the laser characteristics toward the ones of the carbon dioxide laser, i.e., a sharp cutting and removal effect in tissue due to the extremely high energy absorption in water, seems possible.

In contrast to this laser system, however, the light of the 1.32 μm Nd:YAG laser may be transmitted via flexible quartz light guide fibers without extensive energy losses (transmission greater than 90%). For this purpose, quartz fibers with a low hydroxide (OH^-) content are preferable.

Experimental Studies

The first reports on the 1.32 μm laser were published by Frank and Choy and their colleagues, who carried out in vitro and in vivo tests in various tissues with a surgical focusing hand piece (1, 3). In agreement with the previously mentioned physical data they observed an increased vaporization effect using the laser with a wavelength of 1.32 μm. Choy even reported a cutting effect similar to the one of the carbon dioxide laser.

In tests using rabbit stomach, which were preparatory for the clinical application in gastroenterology and were therefore not carried out with the focused laser beam but with an endoscopic fiber transmission, Sander et al. (7) also report an increased vaporization effect with laser light of a wavelength of 1.32 μm in comparison to the standard wavelength of 1.064 μm. However, the results of these tests are in conflict with those performed by Heldwein et al. (4) on stomach tissue of beagles, and our own in vitro and animal experiments in hare's and beef liver. Heldwein et al. described a three to four times higher coagulation effect at the wavelength of 1.32 μm in comparison to 1.064 μm.

Heldwein's group was interested in the potential use of the 1.32 μm laser for endoscopic hemostasis, whereas we tested the new wavelength with regard to the endoscopic palliative treatment of gastrointestinal tumors in vitro and in vivo in have's liver (5).

Under simulated real irradiation conditions, the light guide target tissue distance was 5 mm, and the irradiation time was 3 s. The power output varied between 20 and 90 W in 1.064 μm and 8 and 36 W in 1.32 μm. Our results showed that the 1.32 μm laser is also suitable for the vaporization of tissue. It is to be noted, though, that for pure vaporization of equivalent tissue volumes only about two-

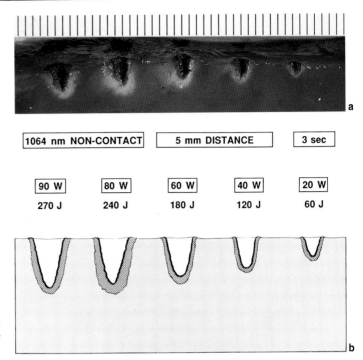

Fig. **1a, b** Tissue effects after a constant irradition time and varying power settings at 1.064 µm wavelength.

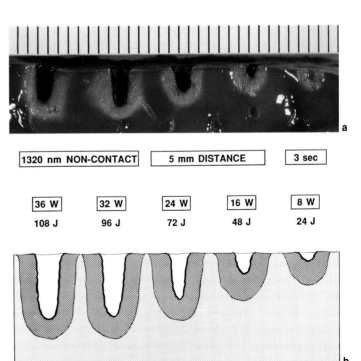

Fig. **2a, b** Tissue effects after a constant irradiation time and varying power settings at 1. 32 µm wavelength.

thirds, and for combined vaporization and co-agulation one-third to half of the total energy are required in comparison to the 1.064 µm laser. Although in the 1.064 µm the coagulation zone surrounding the vaporization defect was always narrower than in the 1.32 µm and widened with the application of higher power settings, this was not the case with the 1.32 µm. Here, we found a very wide coagulation zone in the whole range (8 to 36 W), the size of which was almost independent of the power used (Figs. **1**, **2**).

Clinical Experience

The clinical experience with the 1.32 µm laser in gastroenterology for hemostasis and tumor therapy is limited (2, 6, 7). Sander et al reported favorable coagulation behaviour in endoscopic hemostasis and in the removal of gastrointestinal adenomas. They could not reproduce their observations made in animal experiments concerning an improved cutting capacity of the 1.32 µm laser. Especially in rigid, collagen-rich benign stenoses, they saw unfavorable therapy results. Darker tumor tissue, on the other hand, could be vaporized more effectively, similar to the 1.064 µm laser (7). Sander et al. see possible advantages for the 1.32 µm laser in the removal of tumor tissue with a high water content and in endoscopic hemostasis (6).

In our clinical experience (unpublished data) with a total of 11 patients with gastrointestinal tumors requiring palliative therapy (four esophageal carcinomas, four cardia carcinomas, three colon carcinomas) the laser coagulation effects were greater than in the animal experiments. Vaporization effects were only observed to a low degree. Only if it is possible to increase the energy density at the site of application, will it be possible to achieve sufficient vaporization.

However, the accompanying higher coagulation effect (in comparison to the 1.064 µm laser) will have to be taken into account because it represents an increased risk of complications in palliative tumor therapy with late necroses and resulting perforation.

A clear advantage of the 1.32 µm laser in clinical gastroenterology can at present not be concluded from the available, but only limited, animal experiments and clinical experience. Potential perspectives can be seen not so much in the field of tumor therapy but in the field of endoscopic hemostasis, so that a combination of a high-power 1.32 µm and a 1.064 µm laser in one laser system may be a possibility for the future.

References

1. Choy D, Frank F, Wondrazek F, Rotterdam H, Case R, LaFleur C: Preliminary observations of interaction between several tissues and Nd-YAG laser at two wavelengths. (Abstr 117.) Lasers Surg Med 5: 173, 1985
2. Dwyer R: The history of gastrointestinal endoscopic laser hemostasis and management. Endoscopy 18 (Suppl. 1) 10–13, 1986
3. Frank F, Beck OJ, Häussinger K, Keiditsch E, Landthaler M, Meyer H-J, Unsöld E: Comparative investigation of tissue reaction with 1.06 µm and 1.32 µm Nd:YAG laser radiation. In: Waidelich W, Kieferhaber P (eds): Laser/Optoelectronics in Medicine. Proceedings the 7th International Congress Laser 85 Optoelektronik with 2nd International Nd:YAG Laser Conference. Springer, Berlin: 1986 (pp 290–293)
4. Heldwein W, Lehnert P, Wiebecke B, Ruprecht L, Unsöld E: Investigation of a new 1.32 µm Nd-YAG laser for treatment of bleeding peptic ulcers – Experiments on dog stomach. Lasers Med Sci 2: 189, 1987
5. Hochberger J, Ell C: In comparison 1.064 µm – 1.318 µm Nd YAG continuous wave lasers. In vitro and in vivo experiments with flexible transmission system for tumor therapy in the gastrointestinal tract. Lasers Med Sci. In press
6. Sander R: Neodymium YAG laser therapy of tumours of the lower GI-tract with different wavelength. Seventh Congress of the International Society for Laser Surgery and Medicine, Munich, June 22–26, 1987
7. Sander R, Pösl H, Strobel M, Unsöld E, Frank F, Spuhler A: Nd-YAG Laser in der Gastroenterologie – Erste Ergebnisse experimenteller und klinischer Studien mit der 1,32 µm Wellenlänge. Laser Med Surg 2: 167–171, 1986
8. Stokes LF, Auth DC, Tanaka D, Gray JL, Gulacsink C: Biomedical utility of 1.32 µm Nd:YAG laser radiation. IEEE Trans Biomed Eng 28: 297–299, 1981

General Considerations

Bacteremia After Laser Therapy

B. Kohler, C. Ginsbach, and J. F. Riemann

The occurrence of bacteremia after endoscopic examinations has long been known. The incidence in diagnostic esophagogastroduodenoscopy or colonoscopy is reported to be between 0 and 8% (1, 2, 6, 8). In contrast, after operative endoscopic interventions, such as sclerotherapy of esophageal varices, figures in excess of 50% have been reported (3, 11, 13). It was the aim of the present investigation to establish the bacteremia rate associated with endoscopic laser treatment of stenosing processes within the gastrointestinal tract and its clinical relevance.

Patients and Methods

This prospective study covers a total of 40 patients (17 women and 23 men) with malignant of benign stenosing processes within the upper or lower gastrointestinal tract, in whom a total of 63 laser applications were carried out. The majority of the patients were inoperable because of the advanced stage of the tumor or serious accompanying diseases; a few patients had refused further surgery. Table 1 presents detailed breakdown of the group of patients and indications for laser treatment. The examination was carried out using flexible instruments (GIF XQ 10, CF IBW, Olympus Optical Co.), and a neodymium:yttrium-aluminum-garnet (Nd:YAG) laser (Medilas 2, MBB). Before the examination, the endoscopes were each disinfected for 30 minutes in Gigasept 10%, containing glutaraldehyde, dimethoxytetrahydrofuran, and formaldehyde.

After careful cleansing of the skin, blood was drawn from a vein in the forearm in accordance with the following schedule: immediately before the examination, during treatment with the laser, and 5 minutes, 30 minutes, and 24 hours after termination of treatment. At each scheduled withdrawal, an aerobic and ananaerobic blood culture bottle (BCB System, Roche) was prepared and incubated at 37°C for 10 days. In addition, the leukocytes were counted and the rectal temperature measured before and 24 hours after laser treatment. The following exclusion criteria were used: fever, use of antibiotics within the preceding 7 days, and presence of a central venous catheter or an indwelling bladder catheter.

Table 1 Indications for Laser Therapy

	Patients	Sessions
Endoscopic diagnosis in the upper gastrointestinal tract		
Neoplasms of the esophagus	12	18
Esophagosgastric neoplasms	7	12
Stenosis of esophagogastric anastomosis	1	2
Subtotal	20	32
Endoscopic diagnosis in the lower gastrointestinal tract		
Neoplasms ot the rectosigmoid region	12	19
Stenosing rectal adenomas	5	6
Benign anastomic stenosis	3	6
Subtotal	20	31
Total	40	63

Table **2**   Patients with Positive Blood Cultures

Patient	I	II	III	IV	V	Temperature
Upper gastrointestinal tract						
H. M.	Ø	+ −	−	+	+	Increased sepsis
H. H.	Ø	Ø	Ø	−	Ø	
D. G.	Ø	+ −	+ −	Ø	Ø	
H. M.	Ø	Ø	+ −	Ø	Ø	
B. N.	Ø	−	Ø	−	Ø	Increased sepsis
W. W.	Ø	+ −	−	Ø	Ø	
W. W.	Ø	+	Ø	Ø	Ø	
G. E.	Ø	+	Ø	Ø	Ø	
H. H.	Ø	Ø	+	+	Ø	
W. B.	Ø	+	Ø	Ø	Ø	
J. W.	Ø	+	Ø	Ø	Ø	
Lower gastrointestinal tract						
A. Z.	Ø	+/−	Ø	Ø	Ø	
L. G.	Ø	−	Ø	Ø	Ø	
E. W.	Ø	+/−	Ø	Ø	Ø	
B. S.	Ø	Ø	+/−	Ø	Ø	
J. S.	Ø	Ø	Ø	Ø	−	
E. E.	Ø	Ø	+	Ø	Ø	

+: Aeorbic blood culture
−: Anaerobic blood culture
Ø: Negative blood culture
 I: Blood culture before endoscopy
 II: During laser therapy
III: 5 minutes after laser therapy
IV: 30 minutes after laser therapy
 V: 24 hours after laser therapy

Results

In procedures involving the upper gastrointestinal tract, bacteria were found in the blood cultures in 11 of 32 cases. This corresponds to a bacteremia rate of 34% (Table **2**). In five patients several of the culture bottles proved to be positive. In two cases a positive demonstration of bacteria was accompanied by septic temperatures that required high-dose antibiotic treatment, which, however, failed to prevent the death from septic shock of one of these patients. In the remaining nine cases, the demonstrated bacteremia was of a transient nature and asymptomatic, with no increase in temperature or leukocytosis. The most common organism found was alphahemolytic Streptococcus (Table **3**).

In the lower gastrointestinal tract, the rate of bacteremia was slightly lower at 19% (6 of 31 cases). Here, however, no such complications as fever or sepsis occurred in any of the cases (Table **2**). All cases of bacteremia diagnosed were of a transitory nature and gave rise to no symptoms. The most commonly found organism was Bacteroides species in three cases, followed by Escherichia coli and Staphylococcus aureus in two cases each.

Table **3**   Microorganism and Their Frequency

Upper gastrointestinal tract	
α-Hemolytic Streptococcus	9
Corynebacterium species	5
Bacteroides species	3
Proteus mirabilis	2
Clostridium perfringens	1
Eubacterium	1
Streptococcus faecalis	1
Lower gastrointestinal tract	
Bacteroides species	3
Escherichia coli	2
Staphylococcus aureus	2
Corynebacterium species	1

Discussion

Bacteremia induced by endoscopic procedures has been known since the early days of endoscopy. The first prospective study on this subject was carried out by Le Frock et al. (5) in 1973 who, for rigid sigmoidoscopy, were able to establish a bacteremia rate of 9.5%.

Numerous subsequent studies revealed a bacteremia rate of between 0 and 8% in the case of diagnostic esophagogastroduodenoscopy (1, 2, 6, 8), whereas in the case of endoscopic retrograde cholangiopancreatography, the results vary between 0 and 14% (9, 14), presumably as a function of the endoscopic findings. In the case of sigmoidoscopy or colonoscopy, the current figures vary between 0 and 4% (2, 4, 7, 9). In contrast to these findings, operative endoscopic procedures are associated with appreciably higher rates. Following sclerotherapy of esophageal varices or endoscopic bougienage using Hurst bougies, bacteremia rates in excess of 50% have been observed (7, 10).

Surprisingly, however, only occasional complications, such as fever, occurred and, in the great majority of cases, the bacteremia remained asymptomatic. Relevant complications, such as sepsis or bacterial endocarditis, are absolute rarities (15, 17).

The extent to which endoscopic laser therapy induces bacteremia is a question that, until now, had been the subject of only a single investigation. In the upper gastrointestinal tract, Wolf et al. (16) found a 31% incidence of contaminated blood cultures after laser treatment of malignant tumors in the esophagogastric region.

Our own investigations of the upper gastrointestinal tract revealed an almost identical result. Bacteremia was observed in 34%, being associated with septic temperatures in two serious cases (7%), one of whom died in septic schock despite immediate antibiotic treatment.

In the lower gastrointestinal tract, the incidence of bacteremia was appreciably smaller, namely 19%. In these cases, it was only temporary and asymptomatic. The reason for the markedly higher bacteremia rate in comparison with the purely diagnostic endoscopic procedures is to be found in the marked mechanical irritation of the tumor tissue or mucosa by the endoscope, which promotes invasion by bacteria. In the case of laser treatment within the upper gastrointestinal tract, the most common organisms found were streptococci, corynebacteria, and bacteroides. The latter was the causative organism in the two cases of severe complications.

In laser treatment in the lower gastrointestinal tract, again bacteroides and escherichia coli were primarily found. All these microorganisms are usually saprophytes found within the nasopharyngeal region or digestive tract.

What conclusions are to be drawn from the previously mentioned figures? Is prelaser therapy antibiotic prophylaxis necessary in these, usually immunodeficient, patients?

In 1984, the American Heart Association recommended providing antibiotic prophylaxis in the case of endoscopic examination to be performed in patients with cardiac vitia or who were recipients of artifical heart valves (12). At the present time, we are of the opinion that general routine prophylaxis is not indicated. If, however, fever should occur during the course of laser therapy, immediate broad-spectrum antimicrobial therapy is necessary to prevent further septic complication.

We thank Dr. Dahn and Professor Dr. Fritsche, director of the Institute of Hygiene and Medical Microbiology, Ludwigshafen, for help, advice, and support.

References

1. Baltsch AL, Buhac I, Agrawal A, et al: Bacteremia after upper gastrointestinal endoscopy. Arch Intern Med 137: 594, 1977
2. Botoman VA, Surawicz CM: Bacteremia with gastrointestinal endoscopic procedures. Gastrointest Endosc 32: 342, 1986
3. Cohen LB, Korsten MA, Scherl EJ et al: Bacteremia after endoscopic injection sclerosis. Gastrointest Endosc 29: 198, 1983
4. Dickmann MD, Farrell R, Higgs R et al: Colonoscopy associated bacteremia. Surg Gynecol Obstet 42: 173, 1976
5. Le Frock JL, Ellis CA, Turchik JB et al: Transient bacteremia associated with sigmoidoscopy. Engl J Med 289: 467, 1973
6. Mellow MH, Lewis RJ: Endoscopy-related bateremia. Arch Intern Med 136: 667, 1976
7. Norfleet RG, Mitchell PD, Mulholland BS et al: Does bacteremia follow colonoscopy? Gastrointest Endosc 23: 31, 1976
8. O'Connor HJ, Hamilton I, Lindn C et al: Bacteremia with upper gastrointestinal endoscopy. Endoscopy 15: 21, 1983

9. Parker HW, Greenen JE, Bjork JT et al: A prospective analysis of fever and bacteremia following ERCP. Gastrointest Endosc 25: 102, 1979

10. Raines DR, Brauncke WC, Anderson DL et al: The occurrence of bacteremia after esophageal dilation. Gastrointest Endosc 22: 86, 1975

11. Sauerbruch T, Holl J, Ruckdeschel G et al: Bacteremia associated with endoscopic sclerotherapy of esophageal varices. Endoscopy 17: 170, 1985

12. Shulman ST, Amren DP, Bisno AL, et al: Prevention of bacterial endocarditis. Circulation 70: 1123 A, 1984

13. Snady H, Korsten MA, Weye JD: The relationship of bacteremia to the length of injection needle in endoscopic variceal sclerotherapy. Gastrointest Endosc 31: 243, 1985

14. Stray N, Midtredt T, Valnes K, et al: Endoscopy-related bacteremia. Scand J Gastroenterol 13: 345, 1978

15. Ward RL: Endocarditis complicating ulcerative colitis. Gastroenterology 73: 1189, 1975

16. Wolf D, Fleischer D, Sivak MV Jr: Incidence of bacteremia with elective upper gastrointestinal endoscopic laser therapy. Gastrointest Endosc 31: 247, 1985

17. Yin TP, Dellipiani AW: Bacterial endocarditis after Hurst bougienage in a patient with a benign oesophageal stricture. Endoscopy 15: 27, 1983

Adverse Effects and Complications of Laser Therapy

N. E. Marcon

The application of endoscopic laser therapy in the gastrointestinal tract has expanded in the past 5 years. The initial application of lasers for the control of massive upper gastrointestinal bleeding has been superseded by a newer thrust into endoscopic oncology. This application offers great potential in patient management. Most laser treatments currently are palliative and are carried out in patients who have failed previous therapy by surgery, radiation, or chemotherapy, or in whom serious medical illness precludes traditional surgical modes. Endoscopists are, therefore, faced with difficult clinical problems. These patients are often debilitated and, if they do experience major endoscopic complications, the consequences may be more catastrophic.

A discussion of complications would be remiss if it dealt with percentages only. Also included should be suggestions of improved technique to minimize and avoid complications, as well as to make better patient selections.

Complications

Optic Hazards

Of all the tissue in the body, the retina is the most vulnerable to laser radiation, and an accidental overexposure to a visible or near infrared laser may be catastrophic (see also p. 156). Lesions caused in the retina tend to be thermal. The range of vulnerability of the retina is from 400 to 1400 nm. The seriousness of the clinical effects depends on the strategic location of the laser impulse. If one is so unlucky as to be looking directly into the laser beam at the time of the accident so that a full burn strikes the macula, then the center of vision is destroyed. A burn to the optic nerve can partially or totally destroy the sight of that eye.

In an extensive literature search we do not find any cases of retinal damage in the use of laser in the gastrointestinal tract. This may speak well of the degree of education among laser endoscopists and nursing personnel. One hopes that as laser units proliferate, high standards will be maintained. One can envisage the tendency for error by the laser endoscopist who, distracted by a critically ill patient, fires without suitable ocular precautions. The development of appropriate laser filters that must be electronically in place before the laser is fired, or the construction of endoscopes with built-in, fail-proof lens would offer further protection. The eyes of the patient should also be shielded. Although the low-power helium-neon aiming beam is safe, direct reflection should still be avoided.

The risk of indirect reflection to nonviewing personnel from a internally placed endoscope is remote. The increased use by gastroenterologists of open laser therapy for perianal warts and in protocology renders viewing of the treatment potentially more hazardous. Therefore, all personnel in the endoscopy room should wear protective goggles.

Perforation

The most feared complication of endoscopy is perforation. At times it will be difficult to distinguish whether the perforation is related to the endoscope or to the therapeutic thermal probe – whether it be electocautery or laser light guide.

A high perforation rate with attendant morbidity and mortality, can adversely affect the promising future application of laser endoscopy. The first application of the yttrium-aluminum-garnet (YAG) laser was reported by Kiefhaber et al. (4, 5) for massive gastrointestinal bleeding. Historically, an acceptable perforation rate in these instances would be between 1 and 2% in bleeding patients. Kiefhaber et al's perforations were mainly in acute stress lesions rather than in established, scarred, thick-based chronic ulcers. One factor in the inability adequately to staunch bleeding with thermal laser energy is the heat sink effect of rapidly flowing blood. If the flow can be slowed, coagulation will be promoted with fewer energy impacts and, therefore, a reduced risk of perforation by thermal injury. Mills and Swain (9) have described a coaptive laser probe that accomplishes this with a high degree of success in animal work. Tsunekawa et al. (17) found that sapphire ceramic contact tips have the same effect, but so far have not been the subject of a reported controlled trial. The concomitant use of injection therapy (13) using epinephrine 1:100.000 and 1% polydocanol has been reported by Rutgeerts et al. (12) to reduce blood flow and, therefore, lead to a reduced rebleeding rate and, since less energy is required, a decreased perforation rate.

Coaxial carbon dioxide may lead to painful distension with thinning of the gut wall, especially the cecum, with an increased risk of perforation. This is particularly so in non-contact laser therapy for cecal angiodysplasia. Rutgeerts et al. (11) report a perforation rate of 6% for colonic angiodysplasia but none in laser therapy for gastric angiodysplasia or peptic ulcers. Waitman (19) reports no perforations with argon coagulation of angiodypslasia.

This distension-aggravated complication could be reduced by more careful control of carbon dioxide infusion, better venting, or the use of water-cooled tips.

The presence of pain with free air, fever, leukocytosis is usually an indication for surgery. The so-called benign pneumoperitoneum without other signs of peritonitis may be managed conservatively. Pietrafitta et al. (10) report a perforation rate of 6 of 33 tumors of the esophagus; 5 of these, involving free peritoneal air, were treated conservatively with antibiotics, resulting only in a prolonged hospital stay. The other was a tracheo-esophageal fistula. No site of perforation was determined using contrast material, implying micro perforations with air tracking under pressure from coaxial carbon dioxide. The use of contact sapphire probes to sculpt tumor has resulted in intramural air in the esophagus. The incidence of benign pneumoperitoneum is probably higher than reported, since radiographs are not routinely taken after endoscopy.

Perforation in oncologic situations can be multifactorial. Distortion of the lumen by a large tumor with both intra- and extraluminal spread interferes with proper placement of the endoscope tip and, therefore, the laser shots. This problem may be compounded by previous surgery or radiation therapy. A tumor mass extending outside the lumen may offer some safety as far as perforation is concerned, but usually the functional results are disappointing.

Fistula development occurs usually in the esophagus but could also include the vagina or bladder involvement with rectal carcinoma. Whether these are more related to tumor invasion or concomitant radiotherapy is a moot point. The development of esophago-respiratory tract fistula requires placement of an occluding esophageal prosthesis. Ell et al. (2) report the treatment of fistula into the mediastinum by glue injection. The use of echoendoscopy reported by Takemoto and Hiba (16) may offer some advantage in determining the extent and location of tumor invasion. In those particularly difficult cases with distortion and narrow lumen, current echoendoscopes may be too large. The future development of smaller models will allow better mapping of these tumors with the hope of a reduced risk of perforation. Ell et al. (3) have developed a flexible ceramic coated probe that is passed, like a guide wire, under fluoroscopic control, through a narrow lumen caused by obstructing tumor. The probe acts as a thermal laser-resistant guide and is reusable. It would be ideal for those tumors with a concentric narrowing. In certain extended tumors, rather than persist with repeated treatments, Tytgat et al. (18) suggest that quicker and effective palliation might best be achieved by the earlier use of stents.

In a review of our last 270 patients, five perforations occurred, all in patients with advanced malignant disease. Of 26 patients with obstructing colorectal cancer, one had a perforation. This lesion was in the descending colon in a 64-year-old woman with associated extensive hepatic metastases. She required a resection and terminal colostomy. One of 61 patients with carcinoma of the stomach – a 54-year-old man with obstructing recurrent carcinoma at the gastric outlet – recovered with antibiotic therapy. Of 53 cases of esophageal carcinoma, three had perforation. Two – one midesophageal and one at the gastroesophageal junction – were treated conservatively with antibiotics. The other, with a high esophageal cancer, developed a tracheoesophageal fistula. One month previously, he had completed an unsuccessful course of radical radiotherapy. Death ensued 3 weeks later.

Hemorrhage

It is difficult to ascribe an increased rate of bleeding as a complication to laser therapy alone. The use of the YAG laser in the successful control of actively bleeding upper gastrointestinal lesions is well accepted. Swain et al. (15) report that the laser has been shown to reduce the rebleeding rate in patients who have high-risk stigmata, such as a visible vessel. Occasionally, the laser beam directed at a vessel may lead to vaporizing with either initiation or worsening of hemorrhage.

The usual manner is to rim the vessel in the hope of reducing inflow from the feeding vessel before treating the central vessel. Movement, both respiratory, vascular, or poor endoscopic access, may lead to poorly directed hits and vaporization. In our 23 cases with nonbleeding visible vessels, four cases of fresh uncontrolled bleeding were initiated, and in three urgent operation was required.

Delayed hemorrhage occurs after treatment of both benign vascular lesions or tumor vaporization. In the treatment of angiodysplastic lesions this is decidedly unusual (in 1:64 of our cases). In the treatment of cancers, significant bleeding can occur from trauma by the endoscope or vaporization by the laser. This usually stops spontaneously or with further coagulation. Two patients, one with a fundal carcinoma and the other with rectal carcinoma, had omit requiring transfusion acute bleeding requiring transfusion 4 and 11 days, respectively, after extensive laser coagulation. Both were controlled with acute laser therapy. It is surprising that major hemorrhage is not reported more often.

The use of photodynamic therapy (PDT) in oncology with photosensitizing drugs will be a new frontier for the gastroenterologist in the next decade. The current photosensitizer in clinical use (hematoporphyin derivative

[HPD]; 1) is activated by infrared light in the 630 nm range. The usual source is an argon dye laser. Newer agents may permit the use of wavelengths in the 700 range that allow deeper penetration of light and therefore more tumor destruction. Whether this increased necrosis will result in an increased risk of perforation and hemorrhage remains to be determined. Spinelli et al. (14) report two cases, one gastric and one rectal, with delayed hemorrhage using PDT. The amount of fibrotic reaction in the wall in response to PDT can influence its safety. However, relatively few patients with gastrointestinal disease have been treated. This is a fertile area of future investigation.

Bacteremia

Laser treatment produces vaporization of tissue and these areas of necrosis may serve as an entry focus for bacteria. Tumor treatment also entails trauma to the area by the endoscope and by ancillary dilation techniques, all of which contribute to bacteremia. Kohler et al. (6) do not currently recommend antibiotic therapy for laser therapy on its own account unless there are other conditions in which endoscopy is a risk factor, such as in valvular disease.

Stricture Formation

Laser therapy as applied to most malignant tumors usually does not lead to stricture formation. Seldom is ablation complete for most of these lesions currently referred for laser treatment. Small malignant tumors in the esophagus or near the pylorus could lead to edema or scarring with lumen compromise after successful ablation. The risk is more applicable to benign conditions in the rectum, such as extensive anal condylomata, hemorrhoids, or carpet-type villous adenoma. If the condyloma is extensive, anal stricture is possible, especially if deep ulceration is produced. Hemorrhoidal coagulation is gaining some popularity. If the ulceration produced is excessive, stricture formation and damage to the sphincter is possible. Treatment should be carried out in segmental fashion to avoid circumferential scarring. Mathus-Vliegen and Tytgat (8) have described occasional fibrotic stricture formation in extensive villous adenoma of the rectum in which considerable energy and repeated sessions are required.

Coaxial Gas, General Discomfort

The endoscopic procedure by itself causes a certain amount of discomfort, especially in debilitated patients with obstructing tumors. Distension and discomfort related to laser endoscopy is difficult to quantify and is mainly related to the duration of the procedure with coaxial carbon dioxide. Although absorption of carbon dioxide is more rapid than room air, it nonetheless is a problem. This is especially so with obstructing rectal tumors. The passage of a wire-guided decompression tube as described by Marcon et al. (7) may occasionally be required. The use of contact laser should minimize these problems. Pain related to thermal effect is perceived by the patient in the esophagus and rectum. When the tumor is close to the anal margin, heat generation will produce considerable pain. Pretreatment with a local, long-acting anesthetic to block the perianal area and sphincter will eliminate the discomfort and ensure good sphincter relaxation.

Smoke, Noxious Odours, Viable Viral Particles and Tumor Cell Areosol

Lasers produce their desired clinical effect by the production of heat. This cooking of tissue generates smoke and noxious odors that are distressing to patients and endoscopy personnel. Suitable commercial vacuums with appropriate charcoal filters are available at reasonable cost. The additional use of face mask filters provides further relief. The use of contact probes reduces smoke production. Concerns about aerosols of viable viral or tumor particles caused by vaporization have not been substantiated.

Endoscope Damage

The careless direction of laser beams may lead to damage to outer sheath when shooting with the endoscope sharply turned, as in the rectum or gastric fundus. Direct reflection can lead to damage of the end face of the endoscope. The use of white ceramic hoods will minimize this. The new generation of endoscopes of electronic or CHIP endoscopes have incorporated a shield against laser damage. Injudicious firing of laser while still in the channel will cause damage to the endoscope. Careful attention to good endoscopic technique should overcome these problems.

Summary

Laser therapeutics is entering a new era with great potential for the gastroenterologist. This includes the areas of PDT and gallstone fragmentation. Using appropriate technical skill and clinical judgment, we must realize the great potential benefit of lasers to our patients. However, we must continue our research efforts to improve our results and to avoid complications.

References

1. Dorion DR, Gomer CJ (eds): Porphyrin Localization and Treatments of Tumors. Hess, New York 1984
2. Ell C, Hochberger J, Riemann JF, Lux G: Laser guide for laser treatment of malignant stenosis. Endoscopy 18: 27, 1986
3. Ell C, Riemann JF, Demling L: Endoscopic occlusion of a neoplastic esophago-mediastinal fistula by a fast hardening amino acid solution. Gsatrointest. Endosc 32: 287, 1986
4. Kiefhaber P, Moritz K, Schildberg FW, Feifel G, Herfarth CH: Endoskopische Nd-YAG Laserkoagulation blutender akuter und chronischer Ulzera. (Kongreßbericht 1978) Langenbecks Arch Chir 347: 567, 1987
5. Kiefhaber P, Nath G, Moritz K, Gorisch W, Kreitmair A, Schramm W: Eigenschaften verschiedener Lasertransmissionssysteme und ihre Eignung für die endoskopische Blutstillung. In: Lindner H (ed): Fortschritte der gastroenterologischen Endoskopie. Witzstrock, Baden-Baden 1976 (p 144)
6. Kohler B, Gensbach C, Riemann JF: Bacteremia after endoscopic laser therapy of the upper gastrointestinal tract. (Abstr.) Third Congress of European Laser Association. Amsterdam 1986 (pp. 6–8)
7. Marcon N, Haber G, Kortan P: Colonoscopic decompression of colon in 3 patients with acute pseudo-obstruction using a 10 French nasobiliary set. (Abstr.) Gastrointest Endosc 32: 163, 1986
8. Mathus-Vliegen EMH, Tytgat GNS: Nd-Yag laser photocoagulation in colorectal adenoma. Evaluation of its safety, usefulness and efficacy. Gastroenterology 90: 1865–1875, 1986
9. Mills TN, Swain CP: A coaptive laser fiber endcap to enhance photocoagulation of large diameter vessels. Optopelectronics in Medicine. In: Waidelich W, Kiefhaber P (eds): Proceedings of 7th International Congress with 2nd International Nd. Yag Laser Conference. Springer, Berlin: 1985 (p 351)
10. Pietrafitta JJ, Wei JP, Dwyer PM: Esophageal perforation complicating Nd.Yag laser treatment of esophageal neoplasm. Laser Surg Med 6: 194, 1986

11. Rutgeerts P, Van Gompel F, Geboes K: Long term results of treatment of vascular malformations of the gastrointestinal tract by neodymium Yag laser photocoagulation. Gut 26: 586–593, 1985

12. Rutgeerts P, Vantrappen G, Broeckaert L, Coremans G, Janssens J, Geboes K: A new and effective technique of Yag laser photocoagulation for severe upper gastrointestinal bleeding. Endoscopy 16: 115, 1984

13. Soehendra N, Werner B: New technique for endoscopic treatment of bleeding gastric ulcer. Endoscopy 8: 85, 1976

14. Spinelli P, Andreola S, Marchesini R, Melloni E, Mirabile V, Pizetti P, Zunino F: Endoscopic HpD-Laser Photoradiation Therapy (PRT) of Cancer. In: Porphyrin in Tumor Phototherapy. Plenum Press, New York 1984 (pp 423–426)

15. Swain CP, Bowen SG, Salmon PR: Controlled trial of Nd. Yag laser photocoagulation in bleeding peptic ulcers. (Abstr.) Gastrointest Endosc 30: 137, 1984

16. Takemoto T, Aiba I: Endoscopic ultrasonography in the diagnosis of esophageal carcinoma with particular regard to staging for operability. Endoscopy 18 (Suppl 3): 22, 1986

17. Tsunekawa H, Morise K, Iizuka A, Kanayama K, Furosawa A, Kanemaki N, Hotta M, Daikuzono N: Studies on the application of the newly developed laser microprobes for the Nd-YAG laser endoscopy. Optoelectronics in Medicine. In: Waidelich W, Kiefhaber P (eds): Proceedings of 7th International Congress with 2nd International Nd.Yag Laser Conference. Springer, Berlin 1985 (p 360)

18. Tytgat GMJ, den Hartof Japen FCA, Bartlesman JFWM: Endoscopic prosthesis for advanced esophageal cancer. Endoscopy 18 (Suppl 3): 32–36, 1986

19. Waitman AM: Endoscopic management of vascular abnormalities. In Silver SS (ed): Therapeutic Gastrointestinal Endoscopy. 1 Gaki-Shoin Medical Publishers, New York 1984 (pp 114–129)

Safety Aspects

E. Schröder

Hazards of Medical Lasers

When we discuss the risks of working with medical lasers, we have to distinguish between two different kinds of hazards. The first is due to the hazards of the laser light itself. This is the hazard that we usually think about because we know of the dramatic tissue effects from controlled laser light dosage for desired therapeutic reasons. It is obvious that such effects being applied in an uncontrolled accidental manner can produce damage and thus can cause injury to patients, physicians, or staff members. These damage mechanisms and the rules for preventing them are the main subject of this chapter.

The second potential hazard comes from the laser device itself. To produce laser light, one needs a very complex machine utilizing high voltages, high currents, and sometimes high pressure or toxic gasses. However, we will not discuss these technical risks here, since they are well controlled by government regulations (6).

Hazards of Laser Light

Damage Mechanisms

Instead of producing the desired therapeutic effects, when misused, the laser can be harmful. The different tissue interaction mechanisms can be divided into four categories.

Photothermal Effects. This is the most common damage mechanism. Due to the power of laser light, the tissue is heated by absorption and the result is coagulation, carbonization, or even evaporation. All devices emitting laser light in the visible and infrared region, whether continuous wave (cw) or repetitively pulsed lasers, are able to produce this type of damage.

Photomechanical Effects. Pulsed lasers produce mechanical changes; tissue is torn in different kinds of explosive effects. Although this produces some thermal activity, it is not significant. In fact, the damaged tissue has either a very thin or no coagulation zone, so that bleeding often is an accompanying effect.

Lasers working with very short pulse durations (nanosecond range) mainly produce these effects; but even lasers with microsecond pulses can produce explosive tissue damage if the laser light is absorbed in a small volume.

Photochemical Effects. Low-power laser light below the threshold of thermal effects can cause strong tissue changes by chemical reactions. This is well known from ultraviolet (UV) light effects on skin color. Additionally, photodynamic therapy (PDT) and the controversially discussed biostimulation can also cause photochemical changes. There is also the possibility of mutagenic changes, especially from UV laser light (5).

Please note that the exposure limits given in the following chapter are primarily for thermal and mechanical damage but cannot in all cases be completely accurate, since these mechanisms are not fully understood.

Photoablative Effects. The extreme short UV lines of the excimer laser can produce the so called photoablation. Here, every photon is strong enough to break molecular bonds, so that organic molecules are directly changed to gaseous compounds: solid tissue is thus changed to gaseous products, escaping with high kinetic energy. This is a process of material ablation with very low thermal damage to the adjacent tissue.

From a safety aspect, it is important to consider that a low light dosage, far below the ablation threshold, may have mutagenic potential (5).

Eye Hazards

The eye is that part of a human being that is the most sensitive to laser light and is the most susceptible to irreversible damage.

Table **1** Pathophysiological Effects of Light

Wavelength	Damage to the Eye	Damage to the Skin
UVC (200–280 nm)	Keratitis	Erythema
UVB (280–315 nm)	Keratitis, Cataract	Skin cancer
UVA (315–400 nm)	Cataract	Skin pigmentation, photochemical effects
Visible (400–780 nm)	Thermal and chemical retina damage	Thermal damage, photochemical effects
Infrared (780–1400 nm)	Thermal retina damage	Thermal damage
Infrared (1.4–3.0 µm)	Thermal damage to cornea und lens	Thermal damage
Infrared (3.0–1000 µm)	Thermal cornea damage	Thermal damage

Anatomically, the eye is transparent for visible and near infrared light. The cornea and the crystalline lens, due to their imaging properties, can focus laser light entering the eye to a very small spot size on the retina. The irradiance is thus increased by a factor of 10^5 to 10^6; therefore, even low-power or low-energy levels can lead to partial or even complete damage of the macula.

Table **1** gives an overview of possible damages to the eye; interesting to note is that besides the well-known retina damage of visible light, UV light can be a risk factor in producing a cataract in the crystalline lens. At the other end of the spectrum, mid and far infrared has such a small penetration depth in biologic tissue (corresponding to its high absorption in water), that the laser light cannot penetrate into the eye but produces thermal burns on the cornea.

Skin Hazards

The risk of skin damage is much lower than the risk for the eyes. The damage mechanism is mainly thermal, but one should not forget the photochemical effects, including the carcinogenic potential of UV light.

Table **1** shows these hazards in comparison to those for the eye.

Nonradiation Hazards: Plumes

Several types of surgical laser devices create plumes that contain unpleasant and noxious odors from volatilized tissue components (e. g., the cw neodymium:yttrium-aluminum-garnet (Nd:YAG) laser). Recent publications indicate that there is no hazard from viable tumorous debris (2, 3). Nonetheless, the plumes are sometimes unpleasant and some components may be mutagenic (9). Thus, effective devices for plume removal with proper filters could be useful.

Protection

Classification of Laser Devices

In 1977, The World Health Organization published a schematic for the classification of laser units as a first guideline for users (4). For better understanding, one should know the following physical parameters.

A laser light emission is called a pulsed emission, when the pulse duration is less than 0.25 s. The energy of the pulse is measured in joules. When illuminating an area, the energy density, or fluence (J/cm^2), describes the strength of the light exposition.

In the case of pulse durations greater than 0.25 s, we are talking about cw laser operation. Laser light is measured in energy per time, which is called power (watts). The exposed area is referred to as power density or irradiance (W/cm^2).

Class 1: Non-Risk Laser

The power or energy of the laser light is below the thresholds necessary to produce damage.

The relaxation of control precautions is only for laser light hazards, but care should be taken for technical hazards, such as electricity.

Class 2: Low-Risk Laser

These are lasers of low power, with which an intrabeam viewing is possible but the normal aversion reflex like blinking affords adequate protection.

Two examples are:

Cw lasers emitting in the visible spectrum with power above the maximum permissible power level but below 1 mW.

Scanning laser systems or repetitively pulsed laser in the visible spectrum with power below the maximum permissible power level for an exposure time of 0.25 s.

Class 3: Moderate-Risk Laser

These are lasers of medium power or pulse energy, with which an intrabeam viewing must be avoided. These include the following lasers:

Cw laser from the UV (200 nm) up to the far infrared with maximum power of 500 mW.

Pulsed laser in the same spectral range with a maximum *fluence* of 10 J/cm².

Class 4: High-Risk Laser

In this class not only the beam, but even diffusely scattered laser light can be dangerous. Included are lasers emitting from UV (200 nm) up to far infrared with an average power of more than 500 mW or in the case of pulsed emission lasers, with *a fluence* of more than 10 J/cm².

It is appropriate to remember that all medical lasers, except those for biostimulation, belong to class 4. Several of these lasers working with invisible UV or infrared laser radiation also use an additional visible laser as an aiming beam; this aiming beam can belong to class 1 or 2.

Exposure Limits for Laser Radiation

Laser radiation exposure limits have been recommended in the 1977 WHO report (4). The basic data of the American National Standards Institute (ANSI) 1973 (4) have been incorporated into this list.

Table **2** gives the maximum exposure values at the entrance plane of the eye; many factors were taken into consideration, from the laser beam itself to randomly scattered laser light.

Specific Eye Protection

Today, the most effective eye protection is provided by absorbing filters. These filters can be incorporated into safety goggles, or they can be installed inside the viewing optic of the medical laser device itself, e. g., inside the endoscope, the viewing microscope, or the slit lamp. In this second case it is critically important that the laser light or the illuminated area can only be seen through the viewing optic.

These absorbing filters can be manufactored from plastic or from glass; both are safe against scattered laser light, but not in all cases against the direct laser beam. There have been several accidents with intrabeam viewing with plastic goggles (8) in which the absorbed laser light caused thermal damage to the plastic. Therefore, glass filters are prefered if there is a risk of intrabeam viewing.

Another problem of safety filters is the restriction of color vision. This is not the case when working with invisible UV or infrared laser light; because in this range the goggles are highly transparent in the visible spectrum. When working with the blue-green range of argon laser light, orange-red filter glasses have to be used, or in the case of krypton or ruby lasers, blue filter glasses have to be used.

The worst case is an argon pumped dye laser, which can emit in the whole visible spectrum. Here it is the responsibility of the user to choose the proper safety filter for the actual working wavelength range.

Administrative Regulations

Besides technical protection, such as safety eyewear, and engineering safeguards in the device, such as beam enclosure housings, energy control, and emergency beam-off, there exist several important administrative safety controls that are important for the user; these are the establishment of laser-controlled areas, training of staff, eye examinations, and device maintenance.

Controlled Treatment Area

The ANSI committee has recommended the following safety precautions be incorporated with the use of a controlled treatment area when a class 4 laser is used:

1. Direct supervision by a person knowledgeable about lasers and laser safety.
2. Approval to gain access to the area.

Table **2**   Guideline of Exposure Limits for the Human Eye*

Wavelength (nm)	Exposition Time (s)	Fluence (pulsed lasers) (J/cm²)	Irradiance (cw Lasers) (W/cm²)
UVC 200–280	10^{-2}–$3 \cdot 10^4$	$3 \cdot 10^{-3}$	
UVB 280–302		$3 \cdot 10^{-3}$	
303		$4 \cdot 10^{-3}$	
304		$6 \cdot 10^{-3}$	
305		$1 \cdot 10^{-2}$	
306	10^{-2}–$3 \cdot 10^4$	$1.6 \cdot 10^{-2}$	
307		$2.5 \cdot 10^{-2}$	
308		$4 \cdot 10^{-2}$	
309		$6.3 \cdot 10^{-2}$	
310		0.1	
311		0.16	
312		0.25	
313		0.4	
314		0.6	
UVA 315–400	10^{-2}–10^3	1.0	
	10^3–$3 \cdot 10^4$		$1.0 \cdot 10^{-3}$
Visible			
400– 700	10^{-9}–$1.8 \cdot 10^{-5}$	$5 \cdot 19^{-7}$	
	$1.8 \cdot 10^{-5}$–10	$1.8 \cdot 10^{-3} \cdot Z^{3/4}$	
400– 550	10–10^4	10^{-2}	
550– 700	10–Z_1	$1.8 \cdot 10^{-3} \cdot Z^{3/3}$	
	Z_1–10^4	$10^{-2} \cdot C_B$	
400– 700	10^4–$3 \cdot 10^4$		$10^{-6} \cdot C_B$
Infrared A			
700–1060	10^{-9}–$1.8 \cdot 10^{c5}$	$5 \cdot 10^{-7} \cdot C_T$	
	$1.8 \cdot 10^{-5}$–10^3	$1.8 \cdot 10^{-3} \cdot C_T$	
1060–1400	10^{-9}–$5 \cdot 10^{-5}$	$5 \cdot 10^{-6}$	
	$5 \cdot 10^{-5}$–10^3	$9 \cdot 10^{-3} \cdot Z^{3/4}$	
700–1400	10^3–10^4		$3.2 \cdot 10^{-4} \cdot C_T$
Infrared B + C			
1400– 10^6	10^{-9}–10^{-7}	10^{-2}	
	10^{-7}–10	$0.56 \cdot Z^{1/4}$	
	10		0.1

$C_B = 1$ for $\lambda = 400$–550 nm; $C_B = 10^{0.015\,(\lambda-550)}$. s for $\lambda = 550$–700 nm.
$C_T = 10^{-} \cdot \lambda - 6.4$ nm. $Z_1 = 10 \cdot 10^{0.02\,(\lambda-550)}$. s for $\lambda = 550$–700 nm.

3. Posting of appropriate warning signs.
4. Potentially hazardous beams are to be terminated in a beam stop, whenever possible.
5. Only diffusely reflective materials should be used in or near the beam path (e. g., surgical tools).
6. An emergency disconnect switch.
7. Proper protective glasses available at the entrance to the area.
8. Windows and optical paths that would allow observation of a laser beam should be covered or restricted to reduce the transmitted values of the laser radiation to the nonrisk level.

Training

The training and accreditation of all physicians and staff members who work with medical and surgical lasers has not as yet been strictly regulated, but it is highly recommended. In the near future several government institutes (for example, ANSI) will establish formal requirements for this subject.

Eye Examinations

The present ANSI Laser Standard and the recommendations of WHO state that personnel shall have medical examinations before starting work with medical laser devices. The examination is to evaluate the ocular health of the person and to give a baseline medical record in the event of a suspected exposure above damage thresholds. Routine examinations (once a year) are recommended but not strictly required.

Calibration-Maintenance

It is essential that calibration and maintenance service schedules exist and be followed. Different countries have different regulations on this subject. It is important that protocols cover basic safety checks and that they are required on a strict time schedule (see for example the new German MedGV [7]).

References

1. American National Standard of the Safe Use of Lasers. New York: American National Standards Institute, ANSI Z 136.1, 1973
2. Aronoff BL: Lasers in plastic and general surgery. Med Instrum 17: 415, 1983
3. Bellina JH, Stjernholm RL, Kurpel JE: Analysis of fume emissions after papovavirus irradiation with carbon dioxide laser. Reprod Med 27: 268, 1982
4. Goldman L, et al: Optical Radiation with Particular Reference to Lasers. WHO, Copenhagen 1977
5. Green H, et al: Cytotoxicity and mutagenicity of low intensity, 248 and 193 nm excimer laser radiation in mammalian cells. Cancer Res 47: 410–413, 1987
6. IEC 825: Radiation safety of laser products, equipment classification, requirements and user's guide. 1984. (Corresponding to DIN VDE 0837)
7. Medizingeräteverordnung MedGV, Januar 14, 1985, BGBl I
8. Winburn DC: Laser protective eye wear: How safe is it? Laser Focus, 136–140, April, 1987
9. Wong KC, Oykman PF: Anesthetic consideration in laser surgery. In: Dixon JA (ed): Surgical Application of Lasers. Chicago 1983 (pp 29–40)

Index